T0261916

Memory Games for Groups

Memory Games for Groups

ROBIN DYNES

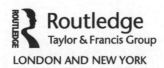

Routledge
Taylor & Francis Group

LONDON AND NEW YORK

First published 1998 by Speechmark Publishing Ltd

Published 2017 by Routledge
2 Park Square, Milton Park, Abingdon, Oxon OX14 4RN
52 Vanderbilt Avenue, New York, NY 10017, USA

Routledge is an imprint of the Taylor & Francis Group, an informa business

British Library Cataloguing in Publication Data

Dynes, Robin

  Memory games for groups

  1. Memory 2. Memory disorders in old age 3. Gerontology – Simulation games

  I. Title

  153.1'2

ISBN 13: 978-0-86388-439-9 (pbk)

Contents

Robin Dynes is a trained counsellor who has worked in the probation service, a number of psychiatric hospitals and private practice. He currently manages a mental health day care centre that provides a wide variety of therapeutic and life-skill groups, including social and creative activities, as well as individual counselling. He has many years of experience in working with groups and with individuals.

In addition to *Memory Games for Groups*, Robin is author the author of *Creative Games in Groupwork* (1988), *Creative Writing in Groupwork* (1990), *The Reminiscence Puzzle Book* (1995), *The Non-Competitive Activity Book* (2000) and *Anxiety Management: A Practical Approach* (2001), all published by Speechmark Publishing.

Introduction

The games in this book, although primarily intended for use with older people, can be enjoyed by people of all ages. They can be used:

- as part of a social activities programme,
- specifically for reminiscence purposes,
- to help keep people oriented to the world around them,
- to exercise memory skills,
- as the prelude to discussion so that individuals can share difficulties and explore methods of aiding memory.

Section 1 provides a guide to using the book and discusses some issues to bear in mind. Suggestions concerning ways to aid memory are also included. These can be introduced into discussions as appropriate when group members share their particular difficulties.

Sections 2–6 each contain 20 games. They are divided into sections to make it easy to find particular games to use for specific purposes. Many of the games can easily be adapted and used under the headings for different sections. The reader should feel free to adapt and use them in this manner. The materials needed for each game are given, together with the preparation required, the procedure, many suggestions for discussion and variations on the theme. Comments are provided which are intended as useful hints about the use of each game.

A feature of the games is their adaptability to the needs of a particular group or individual. Most of them can be made easier or more difficult, as required, and suggestions are offered to facilitate this. Competitiveness has, for the most part, been removed from the games, but can easily be reintroduced, if desirable, by using a points system to produce an individual or team winner.

This adaptability, and the fact that they can be used for fun and enjoyment as well as for more specific purposes, make the games ideal for use in day centres, hospitals and nursing, residential and care homes.

vii

Section One

A Guide to Memory Games for Groups

Issues and suggestions to bear in mind when using the games

USING THE GAMES

One-to-one

A large number of the games within this manual can be used on a one-to-one basis. When working with an individual it is easier to adapt to their pace and develop a strong rapport and trust with them.

Groups

The advantage of working with a group is that one person's memories can trigger off the memories of other group members. They can also share memory difficulties, ways of coping with various situations and possible solutions to problems. Groups also provide a forum which enables people to get to know each other and socialize.

When using the games, ensure that the activity has been adjusted to suit the age, background and experience of the group members or individual with whom it is being used. Adapt the pace and length of time allotted to facilitate concentration levels. Sessions can kept to 10 or 15 minutes and later extended to 20 minutes or longer to accommodate any increase in attention span. Be aware of individuals' ability to hear or see and of any other possible disabilities which will affect attention. If confusion is a problem, a person's memory may be better after they have rested.

REMINISCENCE

There are many gains from reminiscing, including the following:

1 The promotion of self-esteem. Identifying with past achievements and experience can be helpful when people are faced with declining physical and intellectual abilities.

2 Preservation of identity. Being able to hold on to a sense of identity can promote security, which gives strength and motivation to keep going.

3 Stimulation of the traditional role of 'story teller' and preserver of memories. Often people will depict themselves as the central figure or hero in a story worth telling about an event or experience.

4 Reminding people that they have met crises before and have coped with them This can promote motivation to persevere with present demands.

5 Arousal of interest and attention, which enables people to talk about subjects with which they are familiar.

6 Aiding the process of dealing with personal losses and the resulting depression.
7 Helping with the process of reviewing one's life.
8 Enabling the worker to have some understanding of who each person is and how they see the world.

Issues to Keep in Mind

Some caution needs to be exercised when stimulating personal experience. A wide variety of emotions can be triggered, ranging from sadness to happiness, anger to joy and grief to elation. A person can become obsessed with particular past events or situations because of the lack of any satisfactory solution to them and develop feelings of guilt and depression. They may also block the life review process by avoiding certain thoughts and reject the past as a means of avoiding a negative outcome.

Present-day mood may also affect memories. If a person is feeling unwell or down they may look pessimistically on something pleasant which happened in the past. Alternatively, if a person feels well and contented, they may view past experiences, though sad, in a positive way. There may also be conflict between the past and present. Some people need to break with the past and start anew. Others may have already gone through the process of life review and not need to retrace their steps.

The experience of growing older is different for each person and the group leader needs to be aware of and sensitive to these issues. However, for most people it will be helpful to look back.

SHORT- AND LONG-TERM MEMORY

Short-term Memory

Short-term memory can last from a few seconds to a few days and enables individuals to remember long enough to make sense of what is being said in a conversation, or what they read in a book. It allows them to remember what clothes they wore yesterday, what they ate for dinner, what the weather was like or where they put something before breakfast.

Long-term Memory

There is no limit to what can be remembered, no matter what the individual's age, or for how long. This is where information is stored that is required for a

3

long time. Long-term memory enables people to remember what happened to them years before, going back to a time when they were young.

It is likely that, as most people age, there will be some normal reduction in short-term memory, while long-term memory remains intact. This can be very distressing. It is therefore usually most helpful, when working with the elderly, to focus more attention on short-term memory, concentrating on giving lots of reassurance and encouraging the use of aids to memory.

AIDS TO MEMORY

Any aids to memory need to take into account particular individual needs and circumstances. They are likely to be most helpful to those who feel that their memory is failing and are suffering either from normal ageing or from static memory difficulties such as those resulting from head injury or stroke. Some memory difficulties may only be temporary. Causes can include depression, anxiety, emotional upset, isolation and side-effects from drugs.

If memory problems are progressive, as with dementia, strategies can be helpful but need to be regularly reviewed and updated to take account of changing circumstances. Solutions to problems need to be tailored to individual needs. Group discussions can help solve these difficulties. Trying to teach lost skills to someone with progressive problems usually only leads to frustration. It is better to focus on what they can do. Well learned skills and long-standing memory will not normally be affected until impairment is well advanced. Lack of insight may also be a problem. Getting someone to acknowledge that they need to try certain techniques may be difficult.

When the games are used to inspire discussion and exploration of personal difficulties, bear in mind that the group members have been solving their own problems and may have been making use of many memory aids over the years. Sharing and learning from each other is likely to produce the best results.

SOLVING COMMON MEMORY PROBLEMS

It may be helpful to introduce some of the following methods of aiding memory into discussions as appropriate.

Reassurance

Worry and anxiety may be caused by slight changes which occur with ageing, such as an inability to divide attention between several tasks. There may be lack of stimulation because the person is living alone, is less mobile and has become isolated or depressed. Reassurance that no one has a perfect memory and that everyone forgets things from time to time is very important. Also, instead of concentrating on what is sometimes forgotten, it is more useful to reassure by focusing on what people do remember.

Mechanical Aids

These work for appointments, birthdays, anniversaries, as reminders when to make telephone calls, what to do next and assist with remembering what has been said. Mechanical aids include the following:

- wall calendars (gardening, kitchen or hobby memos),
- notice boards (things to be remembered during the day),
- diaries (appointments, birthdays, anniversaries and so on),
- pocket recording cassettes (to recall what has been said),
- alarm clocks (appointment times, when to stop doing something),
- writing pad and pen (by the telephone, the bed, in a handbag or pocket, to write down ideas or things to be remembered).

Remembering Where Things Are

Being organized
This means forming the habit of always returning items to their proper place in each room when finishing with them: cooking utensils to the kitchen, tools to the garage, gardening trowel to the gardening shed, and so on. Something left lying about will, of course, not be where it should be when next needed.

Connection between Object and Place
Put things in places for a reason. Keep garden tools together in the shed, items to do with a hobby in a particular room, and so on.

Labels
Label boxes. All that is needed then is a quick glance at the label to check if that is where the item should be.

5

Lists
Make lists of the places where things are kept. Then, if the person cannot remember where to put something when they have finished using it, the list can be consulted. This list needs to be kept handy, so that little effort is needed to use it. It is helpful to have a copy both downstairs and up.

Going out
Items can be carried in a bag. The bag can be placed in front of the person so that it can be seen at all times. Alternatively, the person can keep in mind the number of items they have with them—umbrella, walking stick, shopping bag and so on. They can then check every now and then to ensure that all the items are there. It is a good idea to put self-addressed labels on items so that they can be returned if they do become mislaid.

Remembering What to Do

Establishing a routine
A good way to aid memory is to establish routines for anything which needs to be remembered. This involves having set days and times for paying bills, going shopping, drawing a pension and so on. This can be reinforced by keeping a brief note in a diary, such as 'pay gas bill', 'do washing' or 'go to day centre'.

Prioritizing
Making lists of things in order of importance that require doing during the day or week can also be useful. People then do what is most important first and end with the least important. If there is too much to do, it can then be decided what can be left for another day.

Remembering at the Wrong Time
Sometimes people remember what has to be done, but at the wrong time or place. If this is a problem, specific times can be set aside each day to reappraise what needs to be done. These need to be times that suit the individual. Good times are before going out in the morning, lunchtime, early evening and before going to bed.

It may suit to reappraise more often, or perhaps less frequently. However, once the habit has been formed, the person is less likely to forget anything.

There are other ways to help remember what has to be done:
- If possible, do things immediately, rather than leaving them.

- If a number of things need to be done, count them and remember how many items there are. Also the person can imagine doing them in order of importance.
- When making a list, items can be written in some meaningful way: items which can be done together, bought in a supermarket, done during the afternoon, in the garden, and so on.
- Attach what needs to be remembered to other daily tasks which are already routine. Examples are taking medication after cleaning teeth, checking a list of things to do at coffee breaks, and so on.
- Repeat what has to be remembered to oneself or speak it aloud several times.
- Set an alarm watch. The person then thinks of what they need to do and associates it with the alarm: when the alarm goes off they will remember what has to be done at that time. Better still, if it can be afforded, is an electronic diary. When the alarm goes off, it will flash a message which has been entered earlier.
- Some people may forget tasks which do not need to be done at specific times. To aid memory, the person can link a task to a time and place and imagine themselves doing whatever it is at the time.
- The person can imagine ridiculous incidents concerning what they want to remember. To remember to buy eggs when they go shopping, they may imagine a giant hen who cannot stop laying eggs: day and night, they keep popping out! When the person passes the eggs shelf in the supermarket this picture will come to mind again and remind them that they need eggs. The more ridiculous the imagining, the better the person will remember.

Prompting Memory

People sometimes experience the feeling that there is something they need to remember, but they cannot recall what it is. If this happens, it may be helpful for them to ask themselves questions appertaining to different areas of their lives: in other words, to classify. Typical questions might be:

- Is it something I have to do before I go out?
- Does it concern my husband or another family member?
- Does it involve anyone other than myself?
- Is it something I have to buy while I'm out?

When people become practised at this they become quicker at tracing what has been momentarily forgotten.

Getting Out and About

Some pre-planning can relieve anxiety about going somewhere. When the person decides where they are going they need to be clear about two things. The first is what they will take with them. They can make a list of items that they will need and check this before they leave. If they are going out to meet someone and do not want to forget something, they can leave the item where it will be seen before they go out—by the front door or in the hall. This needs to be done when it occurs to the person: if they think it can be done later, it is likely to be forgotten.

They also need to be clear about how to get where they are going. Whether they are walking or using transport, a map or a sketch of the route may need to be consulted. The journey can be split into easy stages. It will also be helpful to have written instructions. The person can repeat these aloud and imagine themselves taking the various turnings as they go. As many memory skills as possible need to be brought into play. During the journey, every now and then, the person can picture the route in their mind or repeat the instructions to themselves.

During the journey it is helpful for the person to look at various landmarks so that they will be able to recognize them when returning home. They can also stop occasionally and look back to see what it will look like on the return journey.

Getting Lost

If the person gets lost or takes a wrong turning, it is important not to panic. If they go over the directions again in their mind, it will probably occur to them where they have gone wrong. They can then retrace their steps to that point, or work out an alternative way to get back on their route. If they have done the journey before, they may be able to think of the route they took then; also, there will probably be signposts which can be followed; if not, they can go into a shop and ask directions, or stop someone in the street.

It is a good idea, if they are visiting someone, for them to have that person's telephone number with them so that, if necessary, they can ring them up from a telephone box and ask for directions.

It is important that the person remains calm. They can remind themselves that most people take wrong turnings from time to time. It is not a catastrophe and, usually, it means a delay of only a few minutes. If it is treated light-heartedly and the person remains anxiety-free, it will be easier for them to think and take corrective action.

Remembering People's Names
Being unable to remember people's names can be embarrassing. This should not automatically be blamed on ageing: the person may have mumbled their name when introducing themselves, so that it was not heard properly.

Repeat
The person can be asked to repeat their name. It is then quite natural to repeat the name back to them to make sure it has been heard correctly. If it is an unusual name, the person can be asked to spell it. People like to hear their name spoken so, during the conversation, when addressing the person, the name can be repeated a few times.

Observe
Another way to remember the name is to look at the person. Have they any outstanding features: beautiful eyes, crooked teeth, dimples, gestures, a peculiar manner of speaking or an impish smile? This feature can be exaggerated in the mind, so that the person is imagined with hair trailing 20 feet behind them, arms swirling like a windmill, and so on. As much as possible can be found out about the person: a hobby, what they do for a living, where they live, a piece of scandal, and other details. The more that is known about someone, the more there is to associate with the name.

Reinforce
When trying to remember it is helpful, every so often, for the person to look around the room and observe all the new people they have met. The names can then be repeated in the mind. Also, when saying goodbye or moving on to someone else, the person's name can be repeated aloud: something like "It's been lovely talking to you, William!" or "Goodbye, Jane!" It is helpful to try to recall their name and appearance a short time after leaving the person, and then again a few hours later.

A name diary
If remembering names is a particularly bad problem, a name diary is very useful. As soon as possible after meeting someone, the person's name and a few details about them are written down. This diary can then be kept handy so that it can be referred to quickly. It is acceptable in most circumstances, when meeting someone for the first time, to say: "I must write down your name and address (and telephone number) so I don't forget it." The name and address having been written down, more details can be added later.

9

Be absurd

It can also help to remember people if ridiculous stories about them are made up. The person wanting to remember imagines them doing something heroic, funny or absurd and associates this with them in their mind.

When everything fails

If is important for the person not to panic or feel embarrassed, guilty or stupid if they just cannot remember a name. Reassure them that it is all right not to remember sometimes. It may be helpful to think of the first meeting with the person, where it was, what they were doing and any other details. Along with this information, the name may come back to mind. And if the name still cannot be brought to mind, there are a number of other approaches to try. One way is to be direct, saying something like: "I remember you, but your name has gone right out of my head!" The person will then automatically say their name. Another way is for the person having difficulty to say: "Hello, my name's …", whereupon the other person will almost always reply stating their name. Finally, the conversation can proceed without mentioning names. A statement can be made, such as "It's nice to see you again" and the conversation can continue. Later, when an opportunity arises, someone else who knows them can be asked.

Remembering What Has Been Said

Sometimes remembering what has been said—an instruction, a conversation, a phone message or information to be passed on to someone—can be a problem, but there are ways of getting round this. For example, the person should make sure that what has been said has been understood. They can ask the other person to repeat it or give further explanation until it is understood. If they are being given instructions, these can be broken down into steps. Once the number of steps is known, these can be reviewed, ticking them off one at a time.

Writing down what has been said and then practising remembering it at intervals, by repeating it, may also help. Alternatively, a pocket recorder can be used to a keep a record, with the person speaking the message or summarizing the conversation. This recording can then be played back at intervals.

A third possibility is for the person to think about what they have been told and ask themselves questions about it. Do they agree or disagree with it?

The person could write in a diary or a list of things to do something like: 'Give message to John about …' This will then act as a prompt to the full message.

If the problem is that the person has difficulty recalling something but remembers that they had a message to pass on, they can think of the person who spoke to them. What gestures was the person using when they explained? What were their facial expressions? In what tone of voice was the message given? How did the person feel when the message was given—surprised at first, then angry, or was it relief? Doing this can sometimes trigger what needs to be recalled.

Being reasonable

Ask individuals to give some thought to the fact that, irrespective of age or deafness, something like 40 per cent of the spoken word is not heard or is misunderstood. This is caused by:

- poor pronunciation,
- inaccurate use of words to describe something,
- misinterpretation of words which sound the same,
- bad grammar,
- lack of concentration when listening,
- the speaker not being aware of how much or how little the listener knows,
- hearing what we want or expect to hear and ignoring the rest,
- use of words which have a double meaning,
- what is said is not what is actually meant.

So there is no reason to feel bad or embarrassed about asking for something to be repeated, or for more explanation so that what has been said can be understood; or to feel that the problem is always one of memory or age.

REMEMBERING WHAT IS READ

Newspapers and magazines

If anyone has difficulty remembering what they read, the following formula may be helpful. Suggest they try the following:

1 Read the article or story quickly to find out what it is about.
2 Ask themselves questions concerning what they want to find out about the topic.
3 Read the piece again, this time slowly, looking for the answers to their questions.
4 State—aloud, if possible—what the story or article is about.
5 Repeat the questions they previously asked themselves and decide whether they agree or disagree with the answers provided.

11

It will also help if they discuss what they have read with someone else, repeating the writer's viewpoint and giving their own opinion.

If the person has difficulty later recalling something they have read, they can ask themselves questions such as the following:

Why did I read the article?

What did I want to know?

Did I agree or disagree with it?

Did it have a particular bias or viewpoint?

Was there anything I agreed with?

Did I object to what was being said?

If this fails, they can talk to someone else about the subject. A thought may trigger what they want to remember.

Books

Suggestions to help with remembering the contents of books may include the following:

- Understanding what the book is about before starting to read. This is usually described on the covers.
- Reading the preface or introduction, if there is one, which usually explains the purpose of the book.
- Looking at the contents list and seeing how the subject or story is constructed also noting how it is divided into parts and any other sub-divisions.
- Adapting reading speed to the difficulty of the material: light material can be read fairly quickly; difficult or unfamiliar material will need to be read slowly. If it is a non-fiction book, notes can be made as the person reads.
- Stopping at the end of chapters to think about what has been read and to summarize it in their own words. A good way of doing this is for the person to ask themselves questions about anything they do not understand and then go back and find the answer. By going through this process they will form their own thoughts and relate what they have read to their own experience—and we all remember our own thoughts and experiences best. They will also be sure that they have understood what they have read and will have used repetition to reinforce their memory.
- Discussing what has been read with someone else. If the person does not have anyone to discuss the subject or story with, they can imagine having to recall it and explain it to someone. This also ensures that they understand what has been read and that they use repetition as an aid.

- Reading several books on the same subject. This enables the same information to be repeated in different ways. Any differences in what has been expressed will give more information for the person to form their own opinions on the subject.

Although the individual games in this book can be used for various purposes, their main function is to provide safe frameworks within which people can be helped to stop their memory fading and remain orientated to the world around them while having fun. Keeping the past alive is very important to all of us. To be denied access to memory is also to be deprived of our history and sense of place in the order of things.

Section Two

Personal Memories

Games to help people explore personal memories

2

The Funniest Thing that Ever Happened to Me

MATERIALS None

PREPARATION None

PROCEDURE

Explain that you want each person to think back to a time when something funny or peculiar happened to them. It may have been when they did something silly or frivolous or something that, in retrospect, seems funny. Allow a few minutes for thought, then ask for volunteers or for each person, in turn, to share their event with the group.

Ask each person to describe the experience in detail, including what they were feeling at the time. Stimulate this by encouraging members of the group to ask questions about the event and to share their memories of similar experiences.

VARIATIONS

1 The best thing that ever happened to me.
2 The worst thing that ever happened to me.
3 The most embarrassing thing that ever happened to me.

COMMENT

This is a very pleasant activity to stimulate memory and discussion. People are left with a feeling of shared warmth. Encourage participants to talk about the pleasant or funny side of the events.

Time Machine

MATERIALS Some soft, relaxing music

PREPARATION None

PROCEDURE

Ensure that everyone is sitting comfortably, preferably with their arms resting on the arms of a chair, elbows slightly away from their sides. Start playing some soft, relaxing music. Ask participants to close their eyes and gradually relax as they listen to the music. Tell them to take a deep breath and then let it out with a deep sigh, imagining any tension draining down through their bodies, their legs and into the ground. Do this twice. Now remind them that they are safe and secure.

Allow a brief pause, then say you want them to imagine the room is a time machine which can transport them backwards in time. Is there a time, place or person they would like to go back and visit? It may have been a holiday, a job they did, a house remembered, a garden they cultivated or a person whose company they enjoyed. Give everyone a moment to think and then tell them to imagine that the time machine is transporting them back to that time and place. Now tell them to enjoy the place or talking to the person in their imagination. Allow a few moments' silence for this to happen, then ask everyone to bring their visit to the past to an end and transport themselves back to the present time.

Ask participants to open their eyes, look around, move their arms and feet, say 'hello' to a neighbour and make themselves aware of where they are. Switch the music off and make sure that everyone is safely reoriented.

DISCUSSION

Ask each person to share their visit to the past with the group. Explore where they went and what it was like. Encourage group members to ask questions and explore each individual experience. Discuss why individuals chose a particular place or person to visit. If it was a person, what did they say and what was the outcome?

► *17*

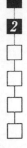

VARIATIONS

1 Have everyone go back to a particular age: 20, 30, 40 or whatever they choose.
2 Have everyone go back to a particular decade: 1950s, 1960s and so on.
3 Have everyone go back to a particular well-known event in the past, such as Queen Elizabeth II's coronation, the assassination of J. F. Kennedy and so on.
4 Have everyone imagine themselves meeting a famous person from the past whom they like or admire.
5 Have everyone visit somewhere in the world they have always wanted to go.

COMMENT

Be aware that some people may feel particularly sensitive to personal memories and may choose not to share them with the group. If this is the case, they may be willing just to say whether they enjoyed the experience. Equally, it could be that particular memory triggers feelings of grief or sadness, and the leader needs to know how to handle this within an open group setting.

However, once one or two people talk about their memories, others usually join in. This exercise can be a very pleasant experience. As people feel secure and relaxed, they usually feel safe about sharing the memory. The important thing is that the person has the memory, even if they do not feel like sharing it.

My Favourite Achievement

MATERIALS None

PREPARATION None

PROCEDURE
Ask members of the group to reflect upon their many achievements in life, such as getting a particular job, bringing up a family, winning at sports, obtaining a qualification, making something, buying a house, helping a friend out, doing something for charity, and so on. It can be something big or small which gave personal satisfaction. Allow a moment or two for thought and then invite each person in turn to share their favourite achievement with the group.

VARIATION
Ask group members to share their proudest moment.

COMMENT
This activity can bring out some real gems. It is good for building self-esteem and a sense of worth for individual achievement.

Personal Adverts

MATERIALS Pens and paper

PREPARATION None

PROCEDURE

Give a pen and a piece of paper to each member of the group. Ask them to write out an advert for themselves as they were at a particular age. Ask them to emphasize their best points. When everyone has finished, have individuals, in turn, read their advert out to the group. Encourage each person to elaborate on what they read out, with other group members asking questions.

DISCUSSION

Have a general discussion at the end about what it was like being the particular age chosen. What are the other group members' memories of it? Again, be aware that this may provoke other emotions, such as regret that their lives are now very different, and make sure there is time to deal with this.

VARIATIONS

Ask group members to write an advert for themselves as:

1 a parent   4 a work colleague
2 a son/daughter   5 a friend
3 a lover or sweetheart   6 a brother/sister.

Add other subjects to this list which will suit your particular group.

COMMENT

To make the game longer and to add more fun, when the adverts have been written collect them and put them in a bag. Then have group members draw them out at random. When each advert is read out, group members try to guess who wrote it.

To make the game less demanding, omit having individuals write the advert; simply have each person in turn describe themselves as they were at their chosen age.

Turning Points

MATERIALS None

PREPARATION None

PROCEDURE

Ask participants to reflect upon their lives and the various turning points there have been. Ask them to think about one in particular: it may be when they decided to leave home, get a job, get married, live abroad, have a career, change jobs, retire, start their own business, and so on. It does not have to be a dramatic turning point—it may be something small which made a difference to the person involved. Ask each person, in turn, to talk about their particular chosen turning point. Encourage them to talk about their life before it and what made them decide to make changes. Perhaps they had no control over what was happening? Then have the person describe how their life was affected afterwards.

DISCUSSION

Have a general discussion about the effects of the turning points. Were there events which seemed disastrous but which, on reflection, turned out to have significant benefits? Do group members have some similar life experiences?

VARIATIONS

Ask the group members to reflect on the way making particular changes in the past has affected them. These could be changes in hair style, how they dressed, eating habits, how they thought about themselves, houses, husbands, wives, moving the furniture around, decorating and so on. Follow the same procedure as above.

COMMENT

This is a good exercise to remind individuals about significant events in their lives. The variation, in particular, lends itself to a lighthearted approach.

What's My Line?

MATERIALS None

PREPARATION None

PROCEDURE
The group can sit in a circle or you could have one member sit at the front facing the others. The individual will have in mind an occupation they have had during their life: carpenter, secretary, housewife, driver, salesperson, motor mechanic, social worker, nurse and so on. The remaining members of the group start asking questions to try to find out what is the occupation. They may only ask questions which can be answered with 'Yes' or 'No'. For example: Did you work indoors? Did you entertain people? Did you sell products? The group are allowed up to 20 questions to find out the correct answer. If the answer is not guessed, have the person state the answer.

DISCUSSION
Give each person ample opportunity to talk about the job before moving on to the next. Explore what doing the job entailed. Did they like doing it? Did other group members do the same or similar jobs?

VARIATION
Ask each person to mime an occupation they have had. The group have to guess what it is from the mime. Questions are not allowed.

COMMENT
To make sure that everyone takes part, have each member of the group ask a question in turn. This game is fun and, as well as stimulating memory, ensures that everyone interacts.

Memory Objects

MATERIALS
A number of mementos, such as a wide selection of postcards, pieces of jewellery, a pen, a scarf, a cigarette lighter, a key, a picture of a house, a picture of a garden, holiday snaps, and so on: the more variety the better

PREPARATION
Place all the items on a table so that they can be seen by everyone

PROCEDURE
Have everyone sit in a circle around the table on which the items are displayed. Tell them to have a good look at the objects (it may be helpful to have them walk around the table to do this). Then ask each person to choose something that reminds them of something from the past. When everyone has chosen an item, they return to their seats with it. Next, ask each person, in turn, to show their chosen item to the group and relate their particular memory prompted by the object.

VARIATION
Ask group members in advance to bring in a personal memento and give it to you without showing it to any other group member. Display the items on a table as before. Ask people to choose an item which is not their own. They then relate their own memory, prompted by the object, and then state who they think owns the memento. When the correct owner has been identified, that person relates their memory associated with the object. The game continues in this manner until everyone has related two memories.

COMMENT
The variation makes the game longer but gives added elements of fun, mystery, observation and more personal participation by group members. Do make sure that everyone gets their possessions back safely.

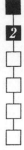

Claim to Fame

MATERIALS   None

PREPARATION   None

PROCEDURE

Everyone has particular characteristics or habits for which they have become well known to family and friends. These may include the following:

baking cakes	a raucous laugh
turning up late	being blunt
being untidy	being kind
organizing everybody	tidying up after everyone
obsession with football	always being early
talking too much	being generous
being superstitious	a sense of humour

Ask group members to ponder about their own particular claim to fame—many may have several. After a moment for thought, give each person in turn an opportunity to share their claim to fame with the group. Encourage them to explain how they came to have the reputation in question and to give examples of it from their life.

VARIATION

Have group members think about and share with the group something in their life at which they have been really good, such as cooking, football, DIY, swimming, gardening, spelling, geography, crossword puzzles and so on.

COMMENT

When people feel safe and able to expose themselves, this can be an enjoyable exercise which brings out both character and idiosyncracies.

Experience Exchange

MATERIALS Pen, paper and a bag

PREPARATION
Write a wide range of experiences down on small pieces of paper—one experience to each piece of paper. Examples:

enviable	kind	festive	boring
annoying	exhilarating	embarrassing	relaxing
military	learning	satisfying	good
sad	adventurous	gourmet	frustrating
rebellious	bad	exciting	jealous
musical	surprising	mysterious	funny
romantic	sporting	spiritual	

Fold the pieces of paper and put them in the bag.

PROCEDURE
Have the group sit in a circle. Now invite each person to draw out a piece of paper from the bag. Allow a moment or two for people to think about the type of experience they have chosen. Someone who chose a musical experience might think back to a time when they went to a concert or a dance, or watched a musical. They then share that experience with the group. Give each member of the group the opportunity to talk about their remembered experience.

VARIATION
To add to the fun, write up different types of experience on a board. Get group members to yell out some of their own. When you have enough written on the board, ask one person to choose an experience to talk about. When their story has been told, that person chooses another experience for someone else in the group to relate.

COMMENT
This is an exercise which can inspire some very unusual stories from the past.

First Time

MATERIALS   Board and chalk

PREPARATION   None

PROCEDURE
Write up on the board a number of firsts. Have group members call out additions to the list. Examples:

First holiday	First meal cooked
First home	First car
First job	First driving lesson
First day at school	First time on an aeroplane
First friend	First date
First boyfriend/girlfriend	First time abroad

When the list is complete, ask each person to think about one of the subjects. When they have done so, invite each group member, in turn, to tell everyone about the first experience they have chosen.

VARIATION
Instead of a list, just give one subject and have each person talk about that particular first experience. Be careful when choosing the subject. It is better if it is one that all group members are likely to have experienced: remember, not everyone may have been abroad.

COMMENT
Some groups can come up with a very long list; too many subjects can be confusing for some or make choosing difficult.

Favourite Things

MATERIALS A pen, pieces of paper and a bag

PREPARATION
Write the names of various favourite things on the pieces of paper—one to each.
Examples:

place	meal	politician
person	country	TV programme
holiday	walk	animal
journey	flower	book
film	mode of travel	song

Now fold all the pieces of paper and put them in a bag.

PROCEDURE
Have the group sit in a circle. Invite members of the group to draw out one piece
of paper each from the bag. If the favourite thing written on the piece of paper is
'a meal', that person thinks back to a meal enjoyed in the past. It may have been
an anniversary dinner, or in an unusual place, or just a type of food thoroughly
enjoyed. The memory is then shared with the group. Encourage other group
members to join in by commenting on their favourite meal. When that subject
has been exhausted, move on to the favourite thing drawn out of the bag by
another group member. Continue in this manner until everyone has had an
opportunity to make a comment on the favourite thing they picked out of the bag.

VARIATIONS
1 Use disliked or hated things: meals, holidays and so on.
2 To keep the exercise shorter, have everyone state and comment on one topic,
   such as their favourite television programme from the past.

COMMENT
Following favourite things with a round of hated things can provide a great deal
of added amusement.

Comparisons

MATERIALS None

PREPARATION None

PROCEDURE

Ask the group members to describe what life was like for them when they were 20 years old. Explore how they felt, what they were doing and so on. After spending some time on this, ask them what life was like when they were 40 years old. Explore this in the same manner and also how they had changed over this period of time. Next, jump another 20 years, to when everyone was 60 years old, and explore this time of life. If appropriate for the group, go up another 20 years and do the same. Compare what it was like being each age.

VARIATIONS

Have the group members compare the following:

1 The experience of living with someone with being on their own.
2 A good year with a bad year.
3 Being a son/daughter with being a parent.
4 Two places lived in.
5 A person liked with a person disliked.
6 A busy time of life with a more relaxed time.
7 A job liked with one disliked.

COMMENT

It will not be difficult to think of many more variations. This is a good exercise to assist with life reviews. However, group leaders need to be aware that painful or sad memories may be evoked by this exercise and they should be prepared to handle this within an open group setting.

Appreciation

MATERIALS Pens and paper; bag

PREPARATION None

PROCEDURE

Give a pen and a piece of paper to each person in the group. Ask them to write down three things that they have appreciated during their life. It could be something someone has done for them, the love of a relative, a kindness, pleasure from music, the companionship of an animal, good health, a sense of humour, an ability to enjoy sport, and so on.

Once everyone has written their three things down, collect and fold the pieces of paper and put them in a bag or bowl. Then ask a member of the group to take one of the papers out of the bag and read it out. Next, everyone tries to guess who the person is who wrote the appreciation list. When the person has been identified, or has owned up, invite them to expand on their three items. Encourage other group members to ask questions and to talk about who or what has been appreciated.

Make it clear to the group that anyone can say "Pass" if they do not want to expand on what they have written. This allows anyone who feels sensitive about a topic to avoid being put on the spot and to maintain their dignity.

VARIATIONS

1 Things I have resented.
2 Things I have found amusing.
3 Things that have puzzled me.
4 Things I have hated.

COMMENT

This exercise can easily be adapted to suit the abilities of group members or to make the game shorter: instead of having people write down what they have appreciated, ask them to think for a moment and then invite them, one at a time, to talk about one or more things in life that they have appreciated.

29

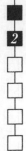

Smells

MATERIALS   Jars and various ingredients

PREPARATION

Put the various smelling ingredients in separate jars. Make sure the jars are covered so that no one can see what is in them. To do this, cover the sides with paper and stretch cloth over the tops or make small holes in tin lids so the smell can seep through. Ingredients might include moth balls, jam, cabbage, lilac, lavender, coffee, lemon, sage, curry powder and hand creams.

PROCEDURE

Ask each person in the group to smell from one of the jars. Ensure that no one says what they think is in the jar. Instead, have each person state a memory associated with the smell: it may be a meal out, a house they have lived in, and so on. To help individuals remember, encourage other participants to ask questions such as: "What sort of house was it?", "Who else lived there?" and "What did you like about it?" When everyone has recounted a memory, have them exchange jars and start the procedure again.

VARIATION

To add extra fun to the activity, number the jars and end the game by having everyone write down what they think the ingredient is in each jar. When this has been completed, invite individuals to call out their answers.

COMMENT

It takes a bit of effort to get all the smells together. However, the activity usually gets a good response and initiates some good discussion about other smells and associated memories from the past.

Life Graph

MATERIALS Pencils

PREPARATION
Photocopy the life graph supplied in Appendix 1: one copy for each member of the group

PROCEDURE
Give each person a life graph and a pencil. Ask them to draw a graph line up or down from the horizontal axis to represent good and bad times over the years. If it was a good time the graph line will rise to good. If it was a bad time the graph line will dive down into the bad section, and so on. When everyone has completed the graph, ask each participant, in turn, to share their graph with the group, telling about some of the bad and good times. Request that everyone ends with a good time.

VARIATIONS
1 When the graphs have been drawn, ask each person to pick out one bad time and one good time to tell the group about.
2 Use the graph to enable individuals to pick out detours, barriers, busy places or major changes experienced to share with the group.

COMMENT
Some individuals may not want to share the whole graph with the group. Suggest they choose one memory from it, good or bad, and share this. This is another good life review exercise.

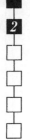

Celebrity Interviews

MATERIALS None

PREPARATION
The amount of preparation depends on group members' abilities. It is useful to prepare a sheet displaying the questions to be asked. This can be given to the people to be interviewed in advance, so that they can prepare answers in their minds. It also gives the interviewer a guide. However, if the group members feel comfortable with it, do the exercise spontaneously without preparation. It is also helpful to have some information about each group member for the celebrity introduction. Alternatively, give the interviewers a few minutes with their subject to discuss how each person will be introduced.

PROCEDURE
Group members can volunteer to be interviewed or instead be encouraged to take a turn, both at interviewing and at being interviewed. Place two chairs so that everyone can clearly see both interviewer and interviewee. The interviewee is introduced as if they are a celebrity. An example would be: "Ladies and gentlemen, we are honoured to have Maureen Webb with us today as our special guest. She is well known for her talent as an artist and her sense of humour." Allow a brief pause for a round of applause. The interviewer then begins the interview, asking questions such as the following:

Where were you born?
What are your memories of childhood?
What was school like?
What was your favourite subject?
Did you have a special friend?
Can you tell us how you met your husband?
What was your first job?

The interviewee answers, giving details about their life. When the interview is completed, the interviewer thanks the person concerned and a round of applause is given.

VARIATIONS

Instead of doing a general interview about each person's life, use specific subjects such as favourite people, hobbies, holidays, favourite television series, cooking, opinions on famous people or past events, friends and so on. Add freely to this list.

COMMENT

To avoid embarrassment or putting individuals on the spot, make it clear before the interviews start that, if anyone does not want to answer a particular question they simply say, "Pass". The interviewer then moves on to the next question.

This activity can provide a lot of entertainment and is useful in helping with life reviews and giving individuals a sense of self-worth.

Tell Me a Story

MATERIALS Paper; bag

PREPARATION
Write a subject on each slip of paper. Examples:

shoes	moving house		
love	cats	dogs	a book
a film	a hobby	being lost	music
games	school	work	shopping
cooking	gardening	decorating	making things
traditions	a party	a relative	eating
misbehaving	children	gossiping	dating
policemen	sport	transport	bad weather
doctors	being late	marriage	

PROCEDURE
Put all the pieces of paper in a bag or hat. Ask each member of the group to draw one out. Give a moment for each person to think about their topic and a story from their own life that is related to it. Give everyone, in turn, an opportunity to tell their story, which can have happened to them or to a friend. If an individual has chosen 'shoes' as the topic, that person tells a story, perhaps about purchasing a particular pair of shoes for a special occasion, or about a pair of shoes they especially liked or disliked.

VARIATIONS
1 Take one subject, write it up on a board, give a moment for thought and then have each person tell their story about the topic.
2 Write a wide selection of topics up on the board and invite individuals to choose their own.

COMMENT
This is a gentle game which often brings out a lot of comic stories and makes remembering fun.

Gifts

MATERIALS None

PREPARATION

Invite participants to bring to the group something that was given to them in the past: this may be an unusual gift, a simple one of little or no monetary value, or one that has sentimental value

PROCEDURE

Place the gifts on a table in the centre of the group so that they can be seen by everyone. When everyone has had a good look, invite a volunteer to talk about their own gift and what it means to them. It may have been given to them for doing someone a good turn, it may have been left to them as a bequest, and so on. Encourage other group members to ask who gave them the gift and what the circumstances were at the time. Questions can be asked about the item itself and the person who gave it. When this has been explored, invite another group member to talk about their gift and go through the procedure again. Continue in this manner until everyone has had an opportunity to tell about their gift.

VARIATION

Invite participants to talk about a special gift they gave to someone else and why it was given.

COMMENT

It is helpful to pass the gift around as the owner talks about it. However, this may not be appropriate if the item is valuable, breakable or the owner objects to this. It is always best to ask permission from the owner first. If the person objects, they may be willing to show the gift to everyone as they talk about it.

The activity can be done without having people bringing the gifts in, but is much more stimulating and effective with the items present.

Satisfying Moments

MATERIALS   Pen, paper and a board

PREPARATION   None

PROCEDURE
Hand out a pen and some paper to each person. Then ask them to write down in a sentence or two a memory of what was a satisfying moment from a particular period in their life. Write the period chosen up on the board; examples:

Childhood (1 to 12 years old)
Teenage years (13 to 19)
Young adulthood (20 to 35)
Mature adulthood (36 to 50)
Older adulthood (51 to ?)

When everyone has written something down about their memory, ask each person, in turn, to share their satisfying moment with the group. They can start by reading out what they have written and then expand on this.

DISCUSSION
Finish the game by writing up all the periods on the board and asking group members what they considered to be the most satisfying period in their life. Explore why and encourage an exchange of memories.

VARIATIONS

Amusing moments	Embarrassing moments	Proud moments
Exciting moments	Lucky moments	Provocative moments
Romantic moments	Unlucky moments	Strange moments
Foolish moments	Dangerous moments	Thrilling moments

Many more topics can be added to this list.

COMMENT

The writing part of the game can be omitted if it is not practical or suited to the abilities of group members. It is, however, helpful to include it if possible.

Of course, all the periods can be written up on a board and then each period in turn can be gone through starting with childhood and finishing with older adulthood.

How Was It?

MATERIALS A board

PREPARATION
Prepare a list of events from a chosen decade, or use the events listed in Appendix 2.

PROCEDURE
Invite members of the group to talk about life in a particular decade of this century. Prompt memories by using the events prepared. Write them up on a board to keep them in people's minds. Either write them all up and have individuals choose one event they remember to talk about or put them up one at a time, inviting anyone who remembers it to comment. Ask what individuals were doing at that time. What was life like then? How old would each person have been? How did life differ then from life now? What have been the main changes in the way people have lived since then? Explore each person's memory of the time as fully as possible.

VARIATIONS
1 Obtain some memorabilia from a particular decade. This can include newspapers, records, postcards, fashions and objects associated with the period. If the actual objects or fashions are not available, you may be able to find photographs in books about the period. Use these to stimulate memories and conversation about life during the decade.
2 Ask the group members to bring in any memorabilia they may have from a chosen decade. This will provide a strong stimulant for personal memories.

COMMENT
In some groups there can be a tendency for participants to focus on the events listed and talk about these exclusively, rather than using them in association with what was happening in their own lives. If desirable, a few carefully placed questions will shift the focus to how the period was for them and what they were doing at the time.

Section Three

The Past

Games to help people exercise long-term memory

Likes and Dislikes	40
Twenty Questions	41
Famous People	43
Activity Mime	44
I Imagine	45
Proverbs	46
Guiding Lights	47
Who Am I?	48
Life Drama	50
True or False	51
Advice	52
Historical Charades	53
Memorable Events	55
Past and Present Debate	56
Memory Browse	58
People Categories	59
Tall Stories	60
Jumbled Novelists	61
Category Shout	62
Seed Sentences	63

39

3 *Likes and Dislikes*

MATERIALS   Pens and paper; bag

PREPARATION   None

PROCEDURE

Choose a particular decade with which members of the group could reasonably be expected to be familiar: the 1940s, 1950s, 1960s, 1970s and so on. Discuss the period briefly, to begin stimulating people's memories. It is important that you do not allow this to continue for too long. Give out the pens and some slips of paper. Ask each person to write down three things they liked and three things they disliked about the period. This could include the music, clothes, hairstyles, people and so on.

When the lists have been completed, collect the slips of paper and put them in a bag. Now have group members, in turn, draw a slip of paper from the bag and read it out. Participants try to guess who wrote the likes and dislikes. When the person has been identified, have them expand on what they have written. Get other group members to add their comments. Continue in this manner until everyone has had their likes and dislikes read out and discussed.

VARIATIONS

Shorten the time needed for the game by leaving out guessing who wrote the comments. If desirable, do not include the decades: simply ask group members to write down three likes or dislikes from the past.

COMMENT

For more able groups, have participants write five likes and five dislikes. For the less able it may be sufficient to have each person call out one like and one dislike. The game is easily adapted to suit any group.

Twenty Questions

MATERIALS   None

PREPARATION

It may be helpful to have a list of famous people from the past ready in case any group members need prompting. Examples: Winston Churchill, Charles Laughton, Rock Hudson, Doris Day, Jane Russell, John Lennon and so on.

PROCEDURE

One member of the group thinks of a person from the past, within living memory, who became famous. It could be a politician, sportsperson, entertainer, explorer or anyone who has done something to become well known. When the participant is ready, other members of the group begin to ask questions in order to find out who is the famous person. Only questions which can be answered with 'Yes' or 'No' can be given a reply. If the group does not guess the answer by the time 20 questions have been asked, they are told the correct answer. Another group member then thinks of another famous person. The group continues in this manner until everyone has had a go.

DISCUSSION

When the correct answer has been revealed, encourage a brief discussion about the famous person. Did people like or dislike them? Why? What do group members remember about them?

VARIATIONS

1   Have participants think of historical characters such as Queen Victoria, Florence Nightingale, Guy Fawkes, George Washington, Buffalo Bill, Billy the Kid, Ned Kelly and so on.
2   Have participants think of characters from fiction. People from books, television and films can be included, such as Chief Inspector Wexford, Miss Marple, Just William, JR Ewing, Huckleberry Finn, Kojak, Crocodile Dundee and so on.

▶   *41*

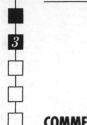

3

COMMENT
This is a game which can also be easily adapted to famous people currently in the news.

Famous People

MATERIALS   Board and chalk or flipchart and magic marker

PREPARATION
Prepare a list of people who were famous during a particular decade of the 20th century, or use one of the lists supplied in Appendix 3

PROCEDURE
Bearing in mind the ages of participants, select a decade from the 20th century and choose the names of a number of people who were famous during the period. Write the names up on a board or flipchart and invite one participant to talk about their memories of the particular famous person they have selected. They may have liked or hated them. Give the person time to express their opinion and then encourage other group members to comment, sharing and exchanging opinions. Explore what the famous person was known for and connect it to what may have been happening in group members' personal lives at that time. Give each group member, in turn, an opportunity to select and talk about one famous person.

DISCUSSION
Finish the activity by having a general exchange of views on what everyday life was like during the chosen decade. What other famous people do participants remember from the same period? Who were their favourites?

VARIATION
There is, of course, no need to stick to just the one decade. Make up a list of famous people from the past and proceed in the same manner.

COMMENT
This activity can stimulate some really good discussions. However, be aware that, while most people are happy to pursue memories of the famous person, a few may not need or wish to explore some memories of their own lives. These may have been particularly sad at that time, or perhaps they find them difficult to deal with now.

43

Activity Mime

MATERIALS   None

PREPARATION   None

PROCEDURE

Call on one person—or ask for a volunteer—to mime a hobby, a job, a sport or other activity they have done in the past. The remaining members of the group have to guess what the activity is. If the group is unable to guess the activity, have the person repeat the mime or mime something else to do with the same job or activity. When this has been guessed, spend a few minutes talking about when the person did it and how long for, and generally explore the memory. Have other group members experience of the same activity? When this has been completed, move on to another volunteer miming a different activity. Continue in this manner until everyone has had an opportunity to take part.

DISCUSSION

End the activity with a general discussion on activities the group members have hated or enjoyed during their lives. Explore why they liked or disliked them.

COMMENT

This is good fun but, in some groups, group leaders may need to help individuals work out how they will do the mime.

I Imagine

MATERIALS None

PREPARATION None

PROCEDURE

Have everyone sit in a circle. One player speaks to another (this can be to the person on their left) and makes an assumption about something that person may have done in the past, starting with the words "I imagine ...". For example: "I imagine you have enjoyed travelling", "I imagine you were a carpenter", or "I imagine you have read a lot of books."

The other person corrects the statement if it is wrong and explains about something they have done in the past. Have the group assist exploration of this by asking questions. Also the person who has made the assumption can say what it was about the person that made them think as they did. When this has been sufficiently explored, the person about whom the assumption was made makes an assumption about the person on their left. The game continues in this manner until everyone has had an opportunity to make an assumption about someone.

VARIATIONS

1 "Did you really believe that ...?" ("Did you really believe that Churchill was the best prime minister ever?"; "Did you really believe that *The Sound of Music* was the best film you have ever seen?")
2 "Is it true ...?" ("Is it true that you were a brain surgeon?"; "Is it true that you were a champion ballroom dancer?")

COMMENT

It is good fun to make a rule that each assumption must be wildly exaggerated or funny. If people have difficulty thinking of things to say, it may be helpful to brainstorm hobbies, occupations and so on, and write them up on a board. This game is fun and gives an opportunity to recall positive achievements and events from the past. The game also lends itself to exploring the present in the same way.

Proverbs

MATERIALS Board (optional)

PREPARATION
Prepare a list of well-known proverbs or use the list supplied in Appendix 4

PROCEDURE
Read out the beginning of a proverb to the group or write the beginning up on a board. Ask if anyone can complete it. Next, explore what the proverb means. For example: 'All that glitters is not gold' means that appearances are deceptive: one should not be taken in by the appearances of people or things. Having established a common meaning, ask group members if they can think of an example from their own lives when they were deceived or knew of someone else who was deceived in this way. Once one person begins, other memories will be prompted. When this topic has been exhausted, move on to another proverb.

VARIATION
Photocopy and hand out to group members the beginnings of proverbs provided in Appendix 5. When everyone has completed the proverbs, have them call out the answers. At this stage explore some of the meanings and have people give examples they have known from life. How many you explore will depend on participants' abilities and the length of time you want the activity to take.

COMMENT
Some proverbs may prompt memories more easily than others in particular groups. If one proverb does not jog memories, move on to another. For some groups, being able to recall the proverb may be sufficient.

Guiding Lights

MATERIALS None

PREPARATION None

PROCEDURE
Ask members of the group to think back to particular people who may have influenced them in a certain way. This could be a famous person, a teacher, a friend, a relative or a stranger. They may have been influential when a decision was made to move house, change jobs, dress in a particular way, leave home, take up a particular career and so on. The influence may be for good or bad.

Allow a few moments for thought and then give each person, in turn, the opportunity to share with the group what it was that made them listen and what was the outcome. Encourage other group members to help them explore their memory of the person who influenced them and of the experience.

DISCUSSION
Close the activity with a general exploration of people who have been major influences on individuals' lives. What else has been a major influence on the way they have lived their lives?

VARIATION
Ask group members to think about some way in which they feel they have influenced someone in the past. Explore this in the same manner.

COMMENT
This activity provides a really strong stimulant for memory.

3

Who Am I?

MATERIALS   Pen, labels, pins

PREPARATION
Write the names of people who have been famous during the living memories of
the people in the group on the labels—one name to each label. Suggestions can
be found in Appendix 6; additional names can be taken from Appendix 3.

PROCEDURE
Pin a label, bearing the name of a famous person, on each person's back.
Request that participants circulate and ask questions of other people to discover
the name attached to their back. For example: "Was I a film star?", "Am I
American?", "Was I in musicals?" or "Do I have blonde hair?"

When answering questions, participants can only answer with a 'Yes' or 'No'.
Individuals keep circulating and asking questions until they discover who they
are.

DISCUSSION
When everyone has discovered who they are, have the group sit in a circle and
discuss the famous people. Who liked or disliked them? What do people
remember about them?

VARIATIONS
1 Use the names of famous couples, one name to each label. Individuals
   circulate until they find their partner. The group then share their memories
   the famous couples.
2 Use the names of actors who starred in particular films or television shows,
   writing the name of the actor on one label and the film or show on another.
   Individuals then match up the film or television show with the actor and
   finish with a discussion about the actor and the film.
3 Use the names of singers and songs in the same manner.
4 Use books and authors.
5 Use people and events.

COMMENT
This game is helpful in breaking down resistance to mixing and talking to other people. It can also be used to pair people up to continue with another game.

Life Drama

MATERIALS None

PREPARATION None

PROCEDURE

Split participants into two or three small groups. Ask each group to think back to when something comic or amusing happened to individuals. It may have occurred at a wedding, while on holiday, at work or at home. When each group has talked amongst themselves about incidents that have happened, they select one and then work out how they can re-enact it, with each person taking a part. It is a good idea for the person to whom it happened to direct the performance.

When all the groups are ready they take it in turns to present a dramatization of their incident for everyone. When this has been completed, the groups can get together again and choose another incident to re-enact. This process continues, if enough time is available, until everyone has had an incident from their lives re-enacted.

DISCUSSION

When everyone has finished performing, bring them back into a circle and give them an opportunity to say how they felt replaying something from their past. Did the presentation reflect how it seemed to them?

VARIATION

Instead of amusing incidents, use achievements, such as winning a sports event being presented with a prize, a silver wedding, winning at bingo, a celebration and so on.

COMMENT

Sometimes people can be reluctant to take part in this activity but, once the fun begins, barriers soon begin to break down. The activity gives an opportunity, not just to tell the incident, but for it to be gone over several times, thus reinforcing the memory of good events and achievements in the past.

True or False

MATERIALS Board (optional)

PREPARATION
Prepare a list of true or false statements concerning well-known people or events that group members could reasonably be expected to remember. Alternatively, use the statements supplied in Appendix 7.

PROCEDURE
Either write each one of the statements up on a board or read it out to the participants. The group members discuss amongst themselves and decide whether it is true or false. When the decision is given, ensure that a true explanation is provided. Also encourage everyone to exchange memories about the event or person.

VARIATIONS
1 Make true or false statements about historical figures or events.
2 Rather than make a statement to the whole group, split participants into two or three smaller groups. Give a few statements to each group, who then discuss them amongst themselves. Allow a set time for this and then bring everyone back together again. Make the statements and have each small group give explanations for the statements they discussed. Then open up the discussion for everyone to be involved.

COMMENT
Statements based on everyday things can spark many memories and discussions.

3 *Advice*

MATERIALS   None

PREPARATION   None

PROCEDURE

Ask each group member to reflect and decide, from their experience of life, what single piece of advice they would give to a person in their teens. Also ask them to reflect on the personal experiences which have made them think as they do.

When participants are ready, have each, in turn, state their advice and say what experiences have influenced that conclusion. When each participant has made their statement, encourage other group members to share their experience concerning the advice. Do they agree or disagree with it?

VARIATIONS

1   What advice do group members wish they had had when they were in their teens and what difference do they think it would have made?
2   What advice did participants receive that has served them well or that they have ignored at their peril?

COMMENT

This is an activity which people can enter into with real enthusiasm and which prompts a lot of memories.

Historical Charades

MATERIALS   Pieces of paper, a pen, a bag

PREPARATION

Write the names of historical characters on different slips of paper. Examples:

Florence Nightingale	Abraham Lincoln	Napoleon
Marco Polo	Guy Fawkes	General Custer
Cleopatra	Christopher Columbus	Queen Victoria
George Washington	Helen of Troy	Rasputin
Karl Marx	Julius Caesar	Oliver Cromwell
Henry VIII	Davy Crockett	William Shakespeare
Joan of Arc	Horatio Nelson	Peter the Great
Thomas Jefferson		

PROCEDURE

Put the pieces of paper in a bag and have a group member draw one out. That person then acts the actual name or does some action relevant to the character's name. The whole name can be acted or the words can be broken down into syllables and each part acted separately until the group has guessed the historical figure.

Before beginning the game do explain the signs the person acting can use to indicate syllables, words or the whole name. They may use noises but should not speak. Alternatively, allow players to speak, but only to say "First syllable", "Second word" and so on.

DISCUSSION

At the end of each act, encourage some discussion on the historical character. What were they known for? What does everyone remember about them? When did they live? Explore as fully as possible.

►

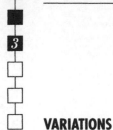

VARIATIONS
1 Use well-known people within living memory.
2 Use film, book or television programme titles.
3 Use places: towns, cities, counties or countries.
4 Have group members think up their own famous people to act.

COMMENT
It can be helpful to have two or three people do one name together, each doing a syllable or a word in a title.

Memorable Events

MATERIALS
Photocopies of old newspaper reports or photographs from books or magazines covering events; board (optional)

PREPARATION
A list of events which have happened during the lifetime of the group members and which they could reasonably be expected to remember; a general list of events is supplied in Appendix 2, but you may be able to add more localized events

PROCEDURE
Call out an event which has happened during the lifetime of the group members or write the event up on a board. If you have photographs or newspaper cuttings about the event, hand these round. After a few moments, ask for a volunteer to share their memory of the event, what happened and what they thought about it. Encourage others to contribute with their own memories adding to the details given. When the subject has been exhausted, move on to another event and proceed in the same manner.

VARIATIONS
1 Use people who have been in the news: politicians, film stars, sports people and so on.
2 Use films and television programmes from the past.
3 Use songs which have been popular.

COMMENT
If you can obtain photographs or newspaper cuttings, these provide a really good stimulus to memory and get the activity going with enthusiasm. It is preferable not to use too many tragic events or disasters.

Past and Present Debate

MATERIALS Slips of paper, pen, bag; board (optional)

PREPARATION
Prepare a list of topics and write one topic on each slip of paper. Examples:

music	children	punishment	entertainment
crime	fashion	courting	weddings
recreation	politicians	sport	customs
community spirit	work	houses	eating habits
education	food	family life	dancing
living standards	health care	travel	cinema
transport	marriage	production methods	

PROCEDURE
Put all the slips of paper in a bag or hat and have one member of the group draw out a topic. That person reads the subject out to the group. Now invite individuals to express their views on the topic. Encourage them to say how they remember it from when they were younger and how they feel attitudes in relation to the subject have changed over the years. How has the subject itself changed over the years? Explore the subject thoroughly. When it has been exhausted, have another group member draw out another topic.

VARIATION
Instead of general subjects, use personal experience topics such as the following:

animals I have owned	cars I have liked
escapes I have had	houses I have lived in
fashions I have liked	jobs I have done
clubs I have belonged to	parties I have attended

Many more themes will come to mind. Discuss, in each case, how attitudes or the subject itself have changed over the years.

COMMENT

Get the group members to call out a list of things which they feel have changed over the years and write them up on a board. When enough topics have been written up, take each subject one at a time for discussion.

Memory Browse

MATERIALS
Old magazines, newspapers and photographs; many of the group may still have old newspapers or magazines they have kept. If you have difficulty obtaining material, packs are available from companies such as Winslow.

PREPARATION Obtain the materials as above

PROCEDURE
Hand out the material you have chosen. Give people time to browse through it. Encourage them to chat about what is in the material. Then ask each person to choose a particular article or photograph that brings back a memory to them. When everyone has chosen, give each participant an opportunity to share their memory with the group. Encourage everyone to ask questions to aid the person telling their story.

VARIATION
Choose a particular theme to discuss, such as records, books, films, fashions and so on, from the period. Use reviews and advertisements from the old newspaper to do this. Who saw the film? What was it about? Who did they see it with? When did they see it? What are the memories of the occasion?

COMMENT
With some groups it may be sufficient to have members look at the papers and magazines. They will automatically start making comments and exchanging memories.

58

People Categories

MATERIALS Pens, paper, board

PREPARATION
Prepare a short list of at least five categories of types of well-known people, such as the following:

politicians	film stars	comedians	singers
rogues	tennis players	footballers	newsreaders
golfers	pop stars	musicians	composers
authors	royalty	fictional characters	

PROCEDURE
Choose five categories or more, depending on how long you want the game to last. Write the five categories up on the board. Give each person paper and pen and ask them to write down three people in each of the categories that they remember during their lifetime.

When everyone has finished this, starting with the first category go round the group members and have them state who they remembered. Ask what is remembered about the famous people. Did they like or dislike them? When the first category has been exhausted, continue in the same manner with the next one, until all the categories have been covered. You will not want to cover every famous person in great detail, only those who seem most popular with the group.

VARIATION
Instead of people, use categories such as world events, films, disasters, television programmes, radio programmes, scandals, books, places visited and so on.

COMMENT
The number of categories can be more or less than five and the number of people to be named for each can be increased or decreased, depending on numbers and abilities of group members. Also, instead of writing the categories on a board, group leaders can write the categories onto the simple category chart supplied in Appendix 8, make photocopies and hand these out to the group.

59

Tall Stories

MATERIALS None

PREPARATION None

PROCEDURE

Ask each group member to think back to something unusual, peculiar or adventurous that happened in the past. It could be something that happened in town they have lived in; it may have happened to a friend or be an achievement, an act of bravery or meeting someone famous; a funny experience or a peculiar hobby someone they knew had; it could be an unusual place visited, and so on. Individuals can choose to tell something which is true or make up a story.

Allow time for everyone to collect their thoughts and then give each person, i turn, an opportunity to tell their story. Once it has been told, other members of the group say whether they think the story is true. The story teller must then ow up and say whether it is or not. Move on to the next player and have that person tell their story. Continue in this fashion until everyone has had an opportunity t tell a story.

VARIATION

Divide the group into teams of three or four people. Each team then chooses a story to tell the whole group. It can be a real story which happened to one of the team, or be made up. Each team member can tell part of the story and the other teams have to decide whether it is true. If it is, they can also try guessing which of the team members it happened to.

COMMENT

This activity introduces a real element of fun. It is extraordinary what people have done or been involved in during their lives.

Jumbled Novelists

MATERIALS   Pens, paper; board (optional)

PREPARATION
Prepare a jumbled list of your own or use the list supplied in Appendix 9;
photocopy whichever list you intend to use

PROCEDURE
Hand out a pen and a sheet of the photocopied jumbled list to each person.
Ask individuals to decipher the jumbled letters which provide the author of each
novel listed. Give sufficient time for everyone to complete the list, then have
group members call out the answers. Alternatively, go round the group giving
each person an opportunity to answer particular questions.

DISCUSSION
Allow time, when answers are being given, for group members to talk about each
book. What was it about? What did they think of it? Alternatively, leave time at
the end of the quiz for a general discussion. Encourage members to talk about
other memorable books and authors they have enjoyed.

VARIATIONS
1   Use films and film stars (list supplied in Appendix 10), songs and singers,
    television programmes and personalities, paintings and artists, sports and
    sports people, musicals and songs, and so on.
2   Use a board to write the jumbled letters on and call out the title of the book.
    Then either the group can call out the author or each person can write the
    answer down.
3   Use the list as a straight quiz, without using the jumbled letters as clues.

COMMENT
This is a quiz-type activity which can easily be adapted to suit participants'
abilities.

Category Shout

MATERIALS Board and chalk

PREPARATION Prepare a short list of categories, such as the following:

composers	footballers	explorers	novelists
royalty	actors	poets	singers
villains	tennis players	politicians	boxers
prime ministers	golfers	presidents	

PROCEDURE

This activity is similar to 'People Categories' but is more easily adapted for individuals with less ability. Write one of the categories up on the board and draw a circle round it. Now invite everyone to call out all the names they can think of in that category. Write these all up on the board as they are called out. When as many as possible have been added to the list, pick one of the names an explore what everyone remembers about that person. What sort of person were they? What did they look like? Were they liked? Encourage the group members t exchange their views and opinions. When one category has been exhausted, move on to another and proceed in the same way.

VARIATIONS

1 Each group member can be asked in turn to name one person in the category and this person is discussed.
2 Call out the category and have the group yell out one name in that category. Then explore as much as possible about that famous person before moving o to another category and another person.
3 Use other subjects such as musical films, books, songs, radio programmes or television programmes in the same manner.

COMMENT

Link memories of the famous person to personal memories of what members of the group were doing at the time in question. This is an activity which can be played at a fast or slow pace to suit the abilities of the group.

Seed Sentences

MATERIALS   Board and chalk

PREPARATION   None

PROCEDURE
Have everyone sit in a circle. Ask each person to think back to when they were young and recall some of things their parents used to say. These may include the following:
Don't talk with your mouth full.
Stand up straight.
Don't drag your feet.
Stop slouching and sit up.
Waste not, want not.
Always be punctual.

Give a moment or two for thought and then have people call out sentences which were characteristic of their early years. Write them all up on the board as they are called out. Also, as each sentence is called out, allow time for individuals to recall and talk about their parents and the incidents which led them to make the remark.

DISCUSSION
When the above has been completed, ask people what influence these sayings have had on their lives. Do any of the sayings still influence them? What sort of things did they say to their own children? Have times changed or do parents still say the same sort of things to their children now?

VARIATIONS
Broaden the topic to include other people in each individual's life, such as brothers, sisters, cousins, teachers, employers, friends and so on.

COMMENT
This can be a very powerful exercise and bring back vivid memories.

Section Four 4

The Present

Games to help people exercise short-term memory and explore ways of remembering things in the present

65

Kim's Game

4

MATERIALS
A tray and a cloth to cover it; pencils and paper; about 10–15 household items. Choose the number of items used and the type according to the abilities of the group members.

PREPARATION Put the household items on the tray and cover with the cloth

PROCEDURE
Seat the group in a circle and place the covered tray on a low table or on the floor so that it can be seen by all. Remove the cloth and ask everyone to make a mental note of what is on the tray. Participants can walk around the tray if they wish to get a better view. When everyone has had the opportunity to have a good look, cover the tray again with the cloth. Now give each person a pencil and a piece of paper and ask them to write down as many of the items as they can remember. When everyone has finished writing, ask each member of the group to call out one item they have written down until all the items have been named.

DISCUSSION
Ask people what methods they used to remember. Did they count the items? Did they classify them by size, shape or colour, split them into stationery or kitchen items, or by some other means? Can the same methods be used to help remember other things such as shopping and other daily tasks participants need to remember? Explore methods used by individuals so that the group can learn memory skills from each other. Group members may also like to express and share their feelings about memory difficulties.

VARIATION
Put into a cloth or plastic bag about 10 small household items, such as a sponge, a ring or a shoehorn, without the group seeing. Pass the bag from person to person, allowing time for each person to have a good feel of the contents within it. When everyone has done this, take the bag away and have participants write down all the items they can remember. When everyone has completed this, have

them call out the objects in turn. As each item is identified, take it out of the bag and show it to everyone.

COMMENT

This is an excellent game to help explore ways of remembering. It can be used with large or small groups and be adapted for use with an individual. When it is used in groups, some people may be tempted to call out items before everyone has had a chance to finish writing. If you do not want this to occur, ask people not to comment.

Who's Missing?

4

MATERIALS None

PREPARATION None

PROCEDURE

Seat the group in a circle. Ask for a volunteer to leave the room. When that person has gone, ask another volunteer to leave the room by another door or to remain behind a screen, so they cannot be seen. Now request that all the players remaining in the group change their position in the circle.

When everyone has settled again, ask the first volunteer to come back into the room. That person studies the group and states who they think is missing. If a player has difficulty identifying the person missing, aid them by asking questions such as: Do you think it is a man or a woman? What is the person wearing? What colour is their hair? Is the person tall or short? If individuals are unable to guess the answers, make it easy by telling them. When the missing person has been identified, have them return to the circle. Continue the game by having another volunteer leave the room, and so on.

DISCUSSION

When everyone has had a go, discuss how individuals remembered. Did they count the number of men and women in the group? Did they note anything else such as clothes worn, colours and so on? Does anyone have particular methods they use to remember? What does it feel like, struggling to remember, and how do people deal with it?

VARIATIONS

1 Send a volunteer out of the room. Instead of asking another member of the group to hide, change something about the group, such as two members exchanging seats, two members exchanging cardigans, or asking someone who wears glasses to give them to someone who does not. Make the change something that can reasonably be spotted. When the volunteer comes back into the room they have to spot the change.

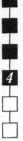

2 Have the person who leaves the room change something about themselves. Perhaps they could change rings from one hand to another, remove a scarf, add a brooch and so on.

COMMENT
If the group members are not familiar with each other, it is a good idea to have a name game before playing. This ensures that everyone is familiar with each other's names. To make the game easier—and the missing person easier to spot—have players remain where they are instead of changing places.

How Observant Are You?

4

MATERIALS
An object such as a biscuit tin, a book, a toy or an ornament; pens, paper

PREPARATION
Write out a list of questions about the object. The following are some sample questions about a tin:

1 What shape is the design on the top of the tin?
2 What colour (or colours) is it?
3 What is it made from?
4 What is written on the lid?
5 What does (or once did) the tin contain?
6 What price is written on it?
7 What is written on the bottom of it?
8 What is the weight of the contents?
9 What is written around the sides?
10 What colour is the rim?

Other questions may be added, depending on the abilities within the group.
If there is a lot of writing on the tin, do not ask questions which require detailed reading.

PROCEDURE
Pass the object around the group, giving each person time to examine it. When everyone has had a good look, place it out of sight. Now give everyone a pen and paper and ask them to write down the answer to each question on your list as you call it out. When this has been completed, go through the questions again. This time have participants call out the answers. Confirm the correct answers by showing the tin or object again.

COMMENT
The activity can be speeded up or made more simple by having group members shout out the answers instead of writing them down.

The Four Seasons

MATERIALS None

PREPARATION A list of seasonal items such as the following:

strawberries	picnics	Halloween	Christmas
falling leaves	ice cream	snow	roses
ice skating	swimsuits	skiing	overcoats
apples	water melon	primroses	air conditioning
tulips	conkers	Easter eggs	holidays
Valentine's day	harvest time	thunder clouds	cherry blossom
lilacs	pantomimes	lambing	Guy Fawkes Night
Brussel sprouts	Mothering Sunday		

PROCEDURE

The group leader calls out the name of something seasonal. This may be a specific holiday, a fruit, an activity or anything else which could be associated with spring, summer, autumn or winter. The participants then reply with the season with which it is associated.

DISCUSSION

Encourage discussion about memories which may be triggered. There will also be disagreements as to whether a certain item is associated with spring, summer, autumn or winter. Open discussion about this is useful.

VARIATIONS

1 Instead of having everyone call out, stipulate that each person has a turn at answering.
2 Use the activity as a team game, with points given for correct answers.
3 Have a brainstorming session, listing what people associate with different seasons of the year.

4

COMMENT

This is an excellent game for orienting individuals' memories to the seasons of the year. However, if you are using the team game variation you will need to make it clear that your decision is final when giving points. Also make clear that the seasonal associations refer to the place where you are playing the game.

Guess Who?

MATERIALS   None

PREPARATION   None

PROCEDURE
Have everyone sit in a circle. To ensure that people are familiar with each other, request that each person, in turn, state their name and say something about themselves that they do not mind sharing with the group. This may be a hobby they have, a favourite colour or a television programme they enjoy. When the round has been completed, allow time for each person to have a good look at everyone else in the group. Now ask for a volunteer to leave the circle and stand with their back to the group. When this has been done, a player in the circle starts describing another member of the group, including the information that person gave about themselves earlier. The person with their back to the circle tries to guess who is being described. When the person has been guessed, another group member has a go at being outside the circle.

DISCUSSION
When everyone has had a go, have a general discussion on the methods people used to remember. Did participants associate different people with something such as a colour, their shape and so on?

VARIATIONS
1 The people in the circle decide which one of them is 'it'. When all is ready, the person outside the circle starts asking questions about the person chosen to be 'it' until they have guessed who it is. Questions can only be answered with a 'yes' or a 'no'. Questions might include: Is this person tall? Is the person a man? Is she wearing a black cardigan? Does she have long hair?
2 Have the player describing the member of the group portray that person in an 'opposite' way, saying, for example, that a thin person is thick-set.

COMMENT
This is a good game for helping people to notice, become familiar with and remember who everyone else is. Encourage humorous and positive descriptions.

73

Truth Game

4

MATERIALS Cards (the same number as there are group members)

PREPARATION Write a question on each card, such as the following:

Which television programme do you like the best?
What has given you the most pleasure during the past week?
What has angered you most during the past week?
Who is your favourite film star?
Which television programme do you dislike the most?
Which domestic chore do you dislike the most?
Which food do you like best?
What is your favourite colour?
Which bad habits annoy you the most?
Which hobby have you tried and really hated?

PROCEDURE
Hand out the cards or have each person choose one at random. Allow a moment for everyone to think about their question. Then ask one person to read out the question on their card and give an answer. Encourage each person to expand on the answer by inviting the other members of the group to ask questions and give personal opinions. When one question and answer have been sufficiently explored, ask another group member to read out their question. Continue in this manner until everyone has answered a question.

VARIATION
Instead of using cards, ask a question and then allow each group member to give their answer to the same question. Encourage the expression of differing opinions and the reasons behind each answer. When one question has been answered and the answers debated, move on to another question. Continue in this manner for the allotted time.

COMMENT
Groups can have a lot of fun with this game. The questions can be varied to suit any group, situation or period of time.

74

What's the Sound?

MATERIALS Tape and tape recorder; pens, paper

PREPARATION
Record a number of sounds of everyday things such as the following:

running water	a tennis ball bouncing against a wall
a car starting	someone playing table tennis
a baby's rattle	someone laying a table
a toilet flushing	someone playing snooker
a vacuum cleaner	someone cleaning their teeth
a cake mixer	a typewriter

PROCEDURE
Give out the pens and paper. Play the first sound and then stop the recording. Allow time for each person to write down what they think the sound is. When ready, play the next sound. Continue in this fashion. When all the sounds have been played, rewind the tape. Ask what the players thought the first sound was. Replay the sound and confirm the right answer. Also take time to explore with the group what it was about the sound that made them recognize it. Does it bring back particular memories? For example, a bouncing tennis ball may bring back memories from childhood or someone's own child playing with a ball. When memories have been explored, move on to the next sound.

VARIATION
Instead of recording the sounds, have some objects such as a baby's rattle, a tambourine, cutlery, a chain, a cake mixer and a tennis ball to hand. Someone can hide behind a screen with the objects and make the sounds for people to write down the answers.

COMMENT
This is another game in which people can shout out the answers, rather than write them down. Also sounds can be very effective in stimulating memories. This game is really good fun.

The Memory Game

4

MATERIALS   Pens, paper

PREPARATION
Prepare a list of questions from a magazine feature article or story which is to be read out. Ensure that the article contains some facts and details, or that the story has quite a few incidents happening in it.

PROCEDURE
Make sure the participants are seated so that they can hear your voice clearly and then read out the chosen piece. Next, hand out a pen and paper to each person. When everyone is ready, begin asking the previously prepared questions. Allow plenty of time for each person to write down the answers. When all the questions have been asked, have group members yell out their answers.

DISCUSSION
When the quiz has been completed, explore with the group the importance of concentration and paying attention in order to remember. This can be stressed by reading out a short piece without telling the group they are going to have to answer questions. Then read out another piece, this time informing them you are going to ask questions. The difference in the amount people remember is usually substantial.

COMMENT
Depending on group members' ability and the time available, it may be quicker and easier to have group members yell out the answers as the questions are asked.

While We've Been Together

MATERIALS   Paper, pens

PREPARATION
Ensure that you have available the same number of pieces of paper as there are people in the group. Write the opening of a statement on each piece of paper. This must relate to the time the group spend together. Examples:

The thing I liked best was ....
The funniest thing was ....
My best memory is ....
The thing which was the least interesting was ....
The thing I'd like to do more of was ....
The person who was kindest to me was ....
The thing I disliked most was ....
The first thing we did was ....

PROCEDURE
Give each member of the group a slip of paper with the opening to a statement written on it and a pen. Allow a moment for thought and then ask each person to write out the completion of the sentence. Then have each person, in turn, read out the whole statement. Encourage them to expand on it by describing the incident or getting other group members' opinions as well.

DISCUSSION
Explore the value of repeating what has gone on in the group and how this reinforces memory.

VARIATION
The above exercise can be used to explore the whole time spent together in a day centre, or to give individuals an opportunity to talk about some things which have happened to them during the past week.

4

COMMENT

This is a good exercise for helping individuals remember the content of the session. The statements can be angled to emphasize and acknowledge the positive experiences during the group's time together.

Earth, Air, Fire and Water

MATERIALS
Board and chalk; a soft object, such as a small, cuddly toy or a sponge

PREPARATION None

PROCEDURE
Have the group sit in a circle. Write the words 'earth', 'air', 'fire' and 'water' up on the board so everyone can see them. Hand the soft object to a player. That person then throws the object to another person and calls out one of the words written on the board. This might be 'air'. The participant catching the object then states the name of a bird, such as a robin or an eagle. If the word called out was 'earth', that person would think of a plant or an animal. In the case of 'water', they would respond with the name of a fish or some type of plant or animal which lives in water. If 'fire' is called out, the person catching the soft object has to remain silent. The player with the object then throws it to someone else, calling out another word chosen from the board.

See how long the process can be kept going without repeating any answers.

VARIATION
Play this as a team game. Line two teams up facing each other. The soft object is tossed to the person opposite, going down the line, then starting back up again.

COMMENT
This is another good quick game which helps with the recall of a wide variety of plants, animals, birds and fish. The game can be slowed down to a quiet pace, with stops to talk about particular animals, plants and so on. The game is also good fun.

Find the Change

4

MATERIALS None

PREPARATION None

PROCEDURE
All the participants sit in a circle. One person leaves the room and changes three aspects of their appearance: for example, taking off a ring, removing or loosening a tie, undoing a button, changing a bracelet from one arm to another, and so on. The person then returns to the circle and the other players say what changes they think have been made. When they have all been spotted, another player leaves the room and makes three changes. The game continues in this manner until everyone has had a go.

VARIATION
1 Split the group into two teams and line them up facing each other. Tell everyone to take a good look at their partner. Then ask everyone to turn, so that teams are back-to-back, and make three changes to their appearance. When the changes have been made, the teams turn to face each other again. Now, starting at one end, have players say what changes the person facing them has made.
2 Have one team leave the room. People then exchange handbags, jewellery, cardigans and so on with their team members. When the teams are brought back together again, each person stands facing the same person as before and spots the changes made.

COMMENT
This is a useful observation and memory game which is good for breaking down barriers.

Whose Face?

MATERIALS Scissors, magazines, paper, pens; board (optional)

PREPARATION
Cut out up to 10 pictures of men and women from magazines (not famous
people) who look quite different. Give the person in each picture a name and
write each name on a separate piece of paper. Also write the appropriate name
on the back of each picture.

PROCEDURE
Place all the pictures on a table with the matching names below them. Ask all the
group members to take a good look at each picture and to memorize the name.
Allow at least five minutes for this. Encourage conversation about each picture
and name. When everyone has had a good look, take away all the names and
change the order of the pictures. Now give each person in the group a pen and a
piece of paper and ask them to write down the name of each person in the
pictures in the new order. When this has been completed, have everyone sit
down and, starting with the first picture, see how many people have succeeded in
remembering and matching the names to the pictures.

VARIATION
To make the game easier, write the names up on a board in a different order
when they are taken away from the pictures. Ask players to match the names to
the pictures.

DISCUSSION
Ask group members what methods they used to help them to remember and
connect the names to the pictures. Did they repeat the name aloud several times
to themselves? Did they remember the names they repeated in conversation
around the table best? Do they do this to remember names when they meet new
people?

Did they make a mental link between the name and the person? If the name
was James Coleman, did they imagine a man sitting eating jam on a pile of coal?
The more unusual the picture they imagine, the more likely they are to ▶

remember the name. Have the group members try doing this with some of the names.

Perhaps there was something unusual about the person in the picture that could be associated with the person's name? Perhaps the person could be linked to someone else who has the same or a similar-sounding name, appearance, occupation, interests and so on.

COMMENT

This is a game which lends itself easily to explaining methods of remembering people and names. It can be used with small or large groups or with an individual. It also encourages people to share their difficulties, thus breaking down barriers and the sense of isolation of individuals with memory problems.

Use a number of pictures suitable to the abilities within the group. For some, four or five pictures may be sufficient; for those who are more able, use 10 to 12.

Colour Call

MATERIALS
An object which can be safely thrown, such as a sponge or a soft ball

PREPARATION   None

PROCEDURE
Have everyone sit in a circle. Throw the sponge to a group member and at the same time call out a colour—any colour you choose. The person who catches the sponge calls out the name of something which is that colour: if the colour called is 'green', the person might say 'grass'. That individual then throws the sponge to another person in the circle and calls out another colour; if the colour is 'red', the catcher might say 'roses'. And so the game continues. Colours may be repeated, but not the answers.

VARIATIONS
Play this as a team game. Line up two teams facing each other. The soft object is tossed to the person opposite, going down the line and then back to the beginning again. See how long it can be kept going without anyone getting stuck.

COMMENT
This is a good quick recall game. It may be helpful with some groups, before starting the game, to have the group yell out as many different colours that they can think of and write them up on a board. Unusual colours can add to the fun and having the colours available can make the game less difficult or threatening for some participants.

Good News

MATERIALS None

PREPARATION None

PROCEDURE
Ask each person, in turn, to share with the group something good that has happened to them during the day or the past week. It can be something big or small. Perhaps someone new spoke to them and they enjoyed the conversation, or they had a favourite meal. They may have received a letter or a telephone call from a friend, or watched a good television programme. Encourage exploration of the event and help individuals to relate a full account of the event and their pleasure.

VARIATION
Bad news can be explored in the same manner as above. However, when doing this, always follow up with a round of good news.

COMMENT
This is a good exercise to help people remember that good things do happen to them. Talking about and repeating such events can help individuals to store these positive happenings in their memory. It is also a very pleasant exercise.

One Minute Test

MATERIALS Soft ball or bean bag

PREPARATION Prepare a list of subjects such as the following:

parts of the body	flowers	shapes	street names
songs	sports	trees	animals
singers	vegetables	films	countries
TV programmes	towns	women's names	makes of car
colours	men's names		

PROCEDURE

Have the group sit in a circle, with a chair in the centre. Have a volunteer sit in the centre with their eyes closed after looking at the list of subjects and choosing one. The others then start passing the bean bag around the circle. When the person in the centre feels ready, they shout out the category they have chosen. The player who is holding the bean bag at that time then names five items from the stated category within one minute. Any player unable to state five items within the minute changes places with the person in the centre.

Encourage other group members to give clues to anyone who has difficulty thinking of items. When the minute is up, start the group passing the bean bag again. After a brief period, the person in the centre of the circle calls out another subject. The game continues in this manner.

DISCUSSION

End the game by having a discussion on the difficulties experienced in recalling some things when required. Explore ways of dealing with this, such as:
- going through the alphabet to trigger words when thinking of the first letter;
- asking the person their name;
- stating your own name to prompt the other person to say theirs;
- always putting things away in their place rather than leaving them where they have been used.

▶ 85

4

COMMENT

This is a game which is good fun and which can help individuals retain their vocabulary and the names of everyday things. The number of items for a subject can be altered to suit abilities within the group.

Word Circle

MATERIALS   Bean bag or soft ball

PREPARATION   None

PROCEDURE

This is a similar game to 'One Minute Test' and is played in the same manner.
Have the players sit in a circle with one person sitting in the middle. This person
closes their eyes and the people seated in the circle pass the bean bag round the
circle. It may go to left or right and change direction at any time. When the
person in the middle feels ready, they call out a letter of the alphabet. The person
with the bean bag at that time then says 10 words beginning with that letter
within one minute. Plurals, proper names and places are not allowed. If the
player states 10 words within the time, the person in the centre closes their eyes
again and the players begin to pass the bean bag again until another letter is
called out. Should any player fail to state 10 words within the time limit, they
change places with the person in the centre of the circle. When players get stuck
for words, have other group members help by giving them clues.

DISCUSSION

End the game by having the group discuss situations in which they have had
difficulty recalling words, names or something. Explore ways of dealing with this,
such as:
• going through the alphabet to trigger a word when thinking of the first letter;
• asking the person their name;
• stating your own name to prompt the other person to say theirs;
• always putting things away in their place rather than leaving them where they
  have been used.

COMMENT

This game can be adjusted to suit abilities. For some individuals, being able to
recall two or three words may be enough. More able groups may find recalling
10 words reasonably easy.

What Do You Remember?

4

MATERIALS
A large poster-size picture or a slide and slide projector; a board; pens, paper (optional). Ensure that the picture or slide has a reasonable number of objects in i

PREPARATION   None

PROCEDURE
Show the slide or picture to the group. Allow enough time for each person to have a good look and observe what is in the picture. Remove the slide or picture and then have the group name everything that was in it. This may include grass, windows, bricks, trees, sky, boats, window sills, shops and so on. Write all the things called out onto a board. When the list is complete, show the picture again and see what has been missed.

DISCUSSION
This is a good game for stimulating exploration of the methods people use to remember. Did they classify items into colour, objects, plants and so on? Did they count the objects? Explore how similar methods can be used to remember everyday things. Encourage the sharing of fears about memory difficulties.

VARIATIONS
1 Have each individual write down a separate list of what they remember.
2 Call out various letters of the alphabet. If there is a picture of a room and you give the letter 'C', participants then write down items such as carpet, chair, coat, cat, ceiling and so on.
3 Ask specific questions about the picture, such as:
   (a) How many people were there in the picture?
   (b) What was the boy doing?
   (c) What colour was the car?

COMMENT
This is an observation exercise which enables the exploration of methods for aiding memory.

Know Your Neighbour

MATERIALS   Small cards, paper, safety pins, pens (optional)

PREPARATION

You will need the same number of cards as there are people in the group. Write up to four tasks on each card. For example: (1) ask No. 2 the name of his/her favourite television programme; (2) find out what is No. 6's favourite meal; (3) what is No. 1's favourite colour?; (4) where was No. 8 born? Also write numbers on small pieces of paper which can be pinned to each person in the group.

PROCEDURE

Ensure that each person in the group has a number pinned to them that is easily seen. Give each group member a card with questions on it and instruct them to circulate and carry out the tasks written on it. Players can, if they wish, make notes of the answers.

When sufficient time has elapsed for everyone to have completed the tasks, have them sit in a circle. Now ask each person, one at a time, to introduce themselves to the group and to say what they have found out about other group members. Any errors of memory can be corrected after each statement is made. This continues until everyone has disclosed what they have found out.

DISCUSSION

To end the exercise, have everyone sit in a circle and explore any difficulties people encountered remembering what had been said to them. What were the causes—perhaps not hearing properly, not understanding the other person, the other person not being clear or feeling nervous and anxious? Explore different ways of dealing with the problems.

COMMENT

The number and type of questions can be adjusted to suit any group. As well as exercising short-term memory, this is a good mixing exercise which ensures people talk to other group members they would not normally approach.

Talk-in

MATERIALS   Music cassette and player

PREPARATION   Prepare a list of topics, such as the following:

royalty	sport	Roseanne	gardening
Home and Away	travelling	Coronation Street	a hobby
fashion	jealousy	The prime minister	art

PROCEDURE
Form the group into an inner and outer circle of equal numbers. Explain that, when the music is playing, the inner circle walks anti-clockwise and the outer circle clockwise. When the music stops, individuals in the inner and outer circle face each other. When you call out a subject, the people in the inner circle talk for two minutes on the topic to the person opposite. When this has been done, the person in the outer circle summarizes briefly what has been said to them ar checks that they have heard correctly. When this has been completed, the music is started up again and the circles walk in opposite directions again until the music is stopped once more. Another topic is called out and this time the outer circle people talk for two minutes and those in the inner circle summarize. Continue in this manner, alternating between the inner and outer circle giving the talk, for as long as is appropriate.

DISCUSSION
Have the group sit in a circle and explore any difficulties people may have had. Discuss the importance of the listener summarizing to check the meaning and accuracy of what has been heard and how this can reinforce memory.

VARIATION
Instead of forming circles, divide the group into As and Bs. People then walk around the room in a random fashion until the music stops. As then find the nearest available B and face them. Continue in the same manner as above, alternating between the As and Bs giving the talk on the topic called out, for as long as is appropriate.

COMMENT

The music adds a sense of fun to this activity which helps participants practise listening and summarizing to ensure they understand accurately what has been said. Listening is an active skill essential to remembering. It involves making an effort but it does improve with practice.

People I Know

MATERIALS   None

PREPARATION   None

PROCEDURE
Have the group sit in a circle. Ask each person to think about someone they know. It may be a neighbour, relative, friend, or someone they would like to know better. They may hate, like, love, despise or admire the person, find them funny or feel indifferent about them. When everyone has had time to think, invite a volunteer to describe what the person they are thinking about looks like. Then have them tell how they came to know the person and explain why they feel as they do about them. Encourage other group members to ask questions about the person being described and to express their opinions. When the player has finished their description and explored the relationship, have another group member do the same. Proceed in this manner until everyone has had an opportunity to speak about a person known to them.

VARIATIONS
1 An odd or peculiar person they know.
2 A member of their family.
3 Someone famous they like or dislike.
4 Their circle of friends.

COMMENT
This activity can bring out some delightful as well as comic stories about people known to group members.

Section Five

5

The World

Games to help people be aware of the world around us

93

Where Am I?

5

MATERIALS None

PREPARATION None

PROCEDURE
Ask each member of the group to imagine themselves in a town or city anywhere in the world. It can be somewhere the person has visited, read about or seen on television. When each person has had time to think of a place, ask for a volunteer to be 'it'. All the other group members then begin asking questions to try and find out the place thought of by that person. The number of questions can be limited to 10, 15 or 20, or left open. Only questions which can be answered with 'Yes' or 'No' can be asked. Examples might include "Is it hot there?", "Does everyone speak French?", "Is it near the sea?", and so on.

Ask people to choose somewhere which other group members might reasonably know. If the group do not guess the answer within the question limit, the person who is 'it' gives the correct answer. The player who gets the answer right has the next go at being 'it', or you could ask for another volunteer.

DISCUSSION
When each place has been guessed, spend a few minutes talking about it. Is it somewhere the player visited or knows well? Who else in the group has been there? What are their memories about it? Did they like or dislike it?

VARIATIONS
1 Limit the places to the country the players live in.
2 Limit the places to the county the players live in.
3 Limit the places to the city or town the players live in.

COMMENT
This is a game which can be varied to keep people familiar with the local area, or to take in the whole world. Do allow some time to talk about the various places, share memories about them, discuss the best time of year to visit them and so on, as appropriate.

94

Geographic Circle

5

MATERIALS None

PREPARATION None

PROCEDURE
Have everyone sit in a circle. One player starts by calling out the name of a place. It can be a town, city, county or country and be anywhere in the world. For example, the player could call out "Manchester". The person next to that person then thinks of another place beginning with the last letter of the place previously stated—in this case the letter 'R'. This player might then say "Rome". The next player then says another place, beginning with the letter 'E'. And so the game continues round the circle. No player can call out a place previously named. If, for example, the letter 'E' came up several times, each player would have to call out a different place beginning with that letter. See how many times the game can be kept going round the circle.

DISCUSSION
End the game by having a discussion about some of the favourite places players have lived in or visited.

VARIATION
Use categories such as flowers, birds, animals, fish and so on. Some of these are more difficult, but you can make them easier by dividing the group into small teams which take turns calling out.

COMMENT
If individual players have difficulty, encourage other group members to help by giving clues without actually stating the place to be named.

Which Flower?

5

MATERIALS Pens, paper, card, glue, magazines, flower catalogues, scissors

PREPARATION
Cut pictures of plants and flowers out of seed catalogues, gardening magazines and so on. Glue them to card and number each one. Make a list of the plant names, making sure that the numbers on the list correspond with the numbers on the cards.

PROCEDURE
Place the pictures on various surfaces around the room. Give each group member a sheet of paper and a pen. Next, tell them to circulate and write down the name and number of each plant or flower. Encourage discussion within the group regarding varieties and so on. The purpose is to get people mixing and talking to help each other.

Allow a set time, depending on the number of pictures, then sit everyone in a circle and, holding up each picture in turn, have players call out the answers. Either go round the group one by one, or have people call out in a random fashion.

DISCUSSION
End the group by giving an opportunity for people to disclose their favourite flower, plant and so on. What sort of gardens have they had in the past? What plants do they grow now?

VARIATION
Instead of flowers use birds, animals, fish, cars, machines and so on.

COMMENT
It takes some initial effort to collect and prepare the pictures for this game. However, once completed, they can be used time and time again. If a number of sets are prepared, they can then be used in rotation.

News Drama

MATERIALS   Newspapers or magazines

PREPARATION   None

PROCEDURE
Split the group members into two or three teams, depending on numbers. Either give each team details about an event in the news from the newspapers or have them select one for themselves. If each team selects an event, ensure that two teams do not choose the same one.

Give the teams time to familiarize themselves with the event and then have them plan a dramatic reconstruction of it. They will need to decide who is going to play which part and who will introduce and do any narrating for the event. When the teams are ready, one team at a time improvises their event for the whole group, who can guess what the event is about. When the improvisation is finished, give a round of applause.

DISCUSSION
After each improvisation, encourage everyone to comment and express opinions about the event and the characters involved. Those who took part in the improvisation may like to make comments, putting the viewpoint of the individual they played.

VARIATION
Use major events from the recent past or from history.

COMMENT
Time spent preparing the improvisation can really help bring out the creativity in individuals. This is a very rewarding activity which is great fun.

The Travelling Game

5

MATERIALS None

PREPARATION None

PROCEDURE
Participants sit in a circle. One person turns to the player on his left and asks, "Where are you going?" The player answers with the name of a city or country. The first person then asks a second question: "What will you do there?" The second player answers, describing something to do with the city or country named. For example:

1st player:	Where are you going?
2nd player:	Paris.
1st player:	What will you do there?
2nd player:	Climb the Eiffel Tower.

The second player then goes through the same procedure with a third player, and so on around the group. See how long it can be kept going without the answers being repeated. If a player gets stuck, allow other team members to help by giving clues to something related to the place named.

DISCUSSION
Finish the session with a general discussion about some of the places named. Many group members may like to share memories of visits they made to them.

VARIATIONS
1 Divide the group into small teams of two or three people. Team members can confer and help each other with the answers. They can also take turns in being spokesperson for their group.
2 To simplify the game, have each person, in turn, call out a place and have the rest of the group state something associated with it. Examples:
   Holland—tulips
   New York—Central Park

5

Dorset—Thomas Hardy
London—Regents Park
Sydney—Opera House

See how long this can be kept going. Places can be repeated, but not the association.

COMMENT
This is a game which promotes quick and imaginative recall.

Current Affairs

5

MATERIALS Pens, paper

PREPARATION None

PROCEDURE
Divide the participants into small teams of three or four people. Give each team
pen and some paper. Instruct them to write down five questions concerning
people or events currently in the news. It is advisable for each team to have a
couple of extra questions in case some of them are similar to those thought of b
the other teams. The group leader can circulate, assisting teams as necessary.
When each team has completed their questions, bring everyone back togethe
again in one big group. Now have each team, in turn, put their questions to the
other group members.

DISCUSSION
Many of the questions will lend themselves to discussion and give an opportuni
for group members to express opinions.

VARIATION
Instead of basing the quiz on current affairs, stipulate that questions be based o
events from the past year, five years, 20 years and so on.

COMMENT
To help people to think up the questions, give teams copies of daily newspapers.
You can also prepare the questions beforehand and have a simple quiz. Howeve
involving group members in making up the questions helps to reinforce current
events more strongly in people's minds.

Ramble

MATERIALS Pens, paper

PREPARATION

Plan a short walk. This may be round the gardens of the building or round the lounge or room in which the activity takes place. Whatever you choose, do the walk and, noting what can be seen and heard, perhaps through windows, prepare a quiz. Questions might include items such as 'What does it say on the board by the front entrance?', 'What colour is the car parked by the side entrance?' or 'What is the gardener doing?'

PROCEDURE

Explain to the group what the planned walk entails and that there will be a quiz when everyone returns. Give clear instructions about where everyone is to go. When participants have completed the planned walk, have them sit in a circle and give them a pen and paper. Now ask the prepared questions, allowing time for answers to be written. When this has been completed, have people call out the answers or go round the group giving each person the opportunity to answer at least one question.

DISCUSSION

End the session with a general discussion. What did people notice that they had not previously observed? Did knowing they were going to be asked questions make them take more notice of their surroundings and thus remember more? What does that tell us about paying attention and memory? Discuss various things people saw, many of which may not have been part of the quiz.

VARIATIONS

1 Instead of having participants write down the answers, have them call them out randomly, giving time to discuss each answer.
2 Give each group member a list of questions to which they must find the answer during the walk.

▶ *101*

5

COMMENT
On a sunny day, this exercise can be really rewarding and give players a great deal of pleasure.

Geography Quiz

MATERIALS   Pen, paper

PREPARATION
Prepare a list of questions about various parts of the world, or use the quiz supplied in Appendix 11.

PROCEDURE
Split the group members into teams. Give each team a pen and some paper and have them appoint a person to write down the answers. When everyone is ready, call out the first question. Allow time for teams to discuss, agree an answer and write it down. When all the questions have been answered in this way, begin going through the answers, with teams calling them out. Alternatively, depending on the ability of group members, have individuals answer the questions.

DISCUSSION
Many group members may have visited, lived in or have knowledge about the various places. As the answers are called out, allow time for comment and sharing of knowledge.

VARIATIONS
1   Base the quiz on the country in which you live.
2   Base the quiz on the county/state in which you live.
3   Base the quiz on your local town, city or area.

COMMENT
This is another game which, once the questions have been compiled, can be used again and again. It is also very useful for keeping people oriented to the area in which they live. The quiz supplied can also be photocopied and handed out to players, if appropriate.

Advertising Slogans

5

MATERIALS   Pens, paper, card, advertisements, scissors, glue; board (optional)

PREPARATION
Cut out about 20 advertisements of well-known products from magazines or other sources. Either blank out or cut off the product names and paste the pictures onto card. Number the advertisements and make a list of the numbers and the corresponding product names.

PROCEDURE
Lay the advertisements on various surfaces around the room. Make sure that they are not in sequence and that players will have to search to find the number they need. Give the participants pens and paper and ask them to list what they think are the product names. Encourage discussion and the exchange of ideas. Allow about 15 minutes to complete the list and then sit everyone down in a circle. Now hold up each advertisement in turn and have the players give their answers.

DISCUSSION
Allow players time to share memories of using each product and their opinions about them.

VARIATIONS
1   To make the activity easier, write the product names on a board or large sheet of paper. Ensure they are not in numerical order. Ask each player to match the product to the numbered advertisements displayed.
2   Give each player a list of prepared advertising slogans. Ask them to look at the displayed advertisements—the product names should not be blanked out for this variation—and write down the product which goes with each slogan.
3   Obtain a variety of advertisements from previous decades and proceed as with any of the variations above.

COMMENT
This is an activity which can be used over and over again. It enables people to move around and mix, and provides fun as well as stimulation for the memory.

Television Expert

5

MATERIALS None

PREPARATION None

PROCEDURE
Seat all the group members in a circle. One player then states: "I enjoy watching [naming a personality and television programme]". The player, having made the statement, then begins to ask each group member one question about the programme or personality. Examples:

What is the programme about?	What time is it on?
Name one actor from the programme.	What channel is it on?
What happened in last week's episode?	
What colour hair does the main character have?	

If anyone is unable to answer a question, open it up to the whole group. When the player has finished asking questions, another player has a go. Continue in this manner until everyone has had an opportunity to ask the questions.

DISCUSSION
After each player has finished asking questions, allow time to discuss and share opinions about the programme selected.

VARIATIONS
1 Films and film stars
2 Books and authors
3 Songs and singers

COMMENT
Depending on the ability of participants, the number of questions to be asked can be varied, with the whole group calling out the answers. This is a good game which refreshes memories about current programmes and stimulates interest in them. It also gives opportunities for players to express opinions about them.

Place to Place

MATERIALS Board, chalk, a reasonable atlas or roadmap

PREPARATION
Choose two well-known cities or places which are far apart; draw a rough outline of the appropriate country on the board and mark the places on the map

PROCEDURE
Have the group sit in a circle, ensuring that everyone can see the board clearly. Ask participants to call out the names of places on the route between the two chosen cities marked on the map. As places are called out, have players mark them on the map. Have an atlas to hand, to check that towns, counties and so on are added correctly. Continue until the map is as complete as possible. After discussion, as outlined below, wipe the board clean and then draw two other well-known cities on a new map and proceed in the same manner once more.

DISCUSSION
Participants may be familiar with many of the places or may have made the journey in question. Explore memories of this and how the places have changed over the years. Discuss other long journeys made by participants.

This exercise can also be used to discuss problems people have in getting from place to place and to share ways of dealing with these problems, including ways of remembering the route, what to do if one gets lost, and so on.

VARIATIONS
Draw a map outline of the main roads in the town, city or area in which participants live. Have players call out various districts, parks, buildings, streets and so on and place them appropriately on the map.

Draw a map of the state or county in which participants live and proceed in the same manner.

To make each variation easier, the names of places between cities, the districts of a town, street names and so on can be supplied by the group leader, so that players then have to mark them appropriately on the map.

▶ *107*

The World

5

COMMENT
Using maps in this way can help to update people on changes which are
happening in local areas and keep them oriented in their own locality.

108

Headlines

MATERIALS A selection of recent newspapers; pens, paper (optional)

PREPARATION
Cut out a range of headlines from the newspapers, or write the headlines in bold print on pieces of paper; keep the original article to which the headlines relate

PROCEDURE
Put all the headlines in a bag. Have a volunteer from the group draw out a headline and read it out. If the player knows what the headline is about, that person then tells the group. If not, ask any other player who knows to inform everyone else. Check for accuracy with the article or give clues to help individuals to remember. If no one remembers, use the article to update everyone. Have group members express opinions on whatever the topic is about. Do they agree or disagree? When the topic has been exhausted, have another group member draw another headline from the bag and continue in the same manner.

VARIATIONS
1 Use photographs from newspapers.
2 To add an element of fun, blank out one or two words in the headlines and place them around the room. Now give each player a pen and some paper and ask them to provide the missing words. When everyone has completed the task, have them sit down and go through the headlines, making sure it is made clear what each headline is about. Many of the substitute words in the headlines will provide much amusement.
3 Use headlines with photographs from articles to prompt memories.

COMMENT
This is an enjoyable way of ensuring that people are made aware of what is happening in the world and have an opportunity to express opinions about it: a good, stimulating exercise.

Jumbled Places

5

MATERIALS Pens, paper; board (optional)

PREPARATION
Prepare a list of jumbled towns and cities or photocopy the list supplied in
Appendix 12.

PROCEDURE
Have the group sit in a circle. Give each person a copy of the jumbled list and a
pen. Ask them to fill in the correct places, using the jumbled letters as a clue.
When this has been completed, have each person, in turn, call out an answer.

DISCUSSION
Round off the game by asking if anyone has visited, has any associations with,
knows anything about any of the places. Explore what group members know
about as many of the places as possible.

VARIATIONS
1 Use places within the country in which players reside.
2 Use places and districts within the county in which players reside.
3 Use places, street names, park names and so on within the town or area in
  which players reside.

COMMENT
To make the game easier for less able participants, write each jumbled place on
board, one at a time, and have the whole group shout out the answer. Discuss
whether anyone has visited or knows the place and then proceed to the next
place name. This is a good game for keeping people familiar with worldwide,
national and local places.

110

I am Going on Tour

MATERIALS None

PREPARATION None

PROCEDURE
Everyone sits in a circle. The first player says, "I am going on tour and will visit Antwerp." The next player says, "I am going on tour and will visit Antwerp and New York." The next player says the two places named plus another of their own choice. And so it continues round the circle.

DISCUSSION
What methods did people use to help them remember? Did they look at each person in turn and associate the place with the person who had named it?

Many of the participants may have lived in or visited some of the places named. Ask them to share their memories of particular places with the group.

VARIATIONS
1 To make the game a little more demanding, make a rule that the first player names a place beginning with A, the second a place beginning with B, and so on. See if the group can complete the alphabet.
2 The first player says, "I am going on a journey and will take an apple with me." The second player adds to the apple another item to take on the journey. And so it continues round the circle.

COMMENT
This game is fun and exercises both concentration and memory.

111

Newspaper Quiz

MATERIALS Several different newspapers

PREPARATION Prepare a list of questions based on what is in the newspapers

PROCEDURE
Have the group sit in a circle. Give each person a newspaper, or part of one. Ask the first question, which might be something like: "What happened in France yesterday?" Each person then searches through their paper to find the article dealing with the question. The person who finds it first reads and explains to the group what has happened in France, or simply reads out the article. Give time for members of the group to comment and express opinions on the incident. When this has been exhausted, move on to the next question.

VARIATION
Split the group into two or more teams. Hand out different newspapers to each group and instruct them to prepare questions. When these are complete, the groups exchange newspapers and, taking turns, start asking each other questions.

COMMENT
This game introduces an element of fun into reminding members about events happening in the world. Magazines can also be used in the same way.

Video Quiz

MATERIALS A television, video and video recorder

PREPARATION
Record a short current affairs, news or other programme about something happening in the world today—this could include drama programmes about current issues. Prepare questions about the programme. Make sure the questions are open-ended and cannot be answered with a simple "Yes" or "No".

PROCEDURE
Show the programme to the group and then ask the prepared questions. Once someone has given an answer, stimulate discussion by asking other members for their opinions on the issue. When the topic has been exhausted, move on to the next question.

DISCUSSION
When the quiz has been completed, ask group members if they remember similar events to that shown in the programme happening in the past. What were the solutions then? Have there been any changes? What is different now? In what way have attitudes changed?

VARIATION
Once the video has been watched, split everyone into two groups who then prepare questions to ask each other about the programme. However, when doing this, be prepared, if necessary, to rerun parts of the video if any disputes arise about the content.

COMMENT
This is a really good exercise for stimulating meaningful discussion about current issues and events.

Famous Places

5

MATERIALS Magazines, travel brochures, scissors, glue, card, pens, paper

PREPARATION
Cut pictures out of the magazines or travel brochures of famous or familiar places such as the Taj Mahal, the Pyramids, the Eiffel Tower, the White House and so on. Paste these onto card, number them and make a list of the places.

PROCEDURE
Lay out the numbered pictures on tables around the room. Give group members pens and paper. Tell them to walk around and look at the pictures, writing down all the places they recognize. Encourage discussion and comments as people circulate. When everyone has written down as many places as they can, have everyone sit down in a circle. Collect the place cards and, holding them up so th the group can see, have the answers called out.

DISCUSSION
Pause when going through the answers to give group members time to commen on the various places. Some may have visited or be able to share information about the places. Alternatively, allow time to do this when all the answers have been given.

VARIATIONS
Use pictures of:
1 famous events
2 birds
3 animals
4 local places such as cinemas, gardens, streets, buildings and historical place of interest.

5

COMMENT

Many variations of this game can be made up, kept and used time and time again so that it becomes a permanent resource. To make it easier for those who are less able, split the group up into small teams of two, three or four people. If mobility is a problem, pass the pictures round one at a time. This is a really useful game.

Categories

MATERIALS
Pens and a photocopy of Appendix 13 (p176) for each player; board (optional)

PREPARATION None

PROCEDURE
Have the players decide on about 10 categories. Each person writes these down in a list, as shown in the first column of Figure 1 below. Someone then chooses letter of the alphabet. Players think of a word beginning with that letter for each category and then write it down, as shown in column 2. Each person tries to think of unusual words which none of the others will have chosen. When everyone has completed the list, or an allotted time is up, players call out their words. Ten points can be awarded for words not used by other players and five points when two or more people have the same word. Once players have counted up their scores and a winner has been established, another letter of the alphabet can be called out. Players now write down words beginning with that letter for each category, as shown in column 3. And so the game continues for as many rounds as are desirable.

Category	C	P	S
FISH	cod	pike	
FLOWERS	carnation	primrose	
CITIES	Copenhagen	Prague	
VEGETABLES	cucumber	parsnip	
COUNTRIES	Cyprus	Poland	
ANIMALS	cow	pony	
COLOURS	cream	pink	
BIRDS	curlew	pigeon	
BOYS' NAMES	Charles	Peter	
GIRLS' NAMES	Charlotte	Patricia	

| *Column 1* | *Column 2* | *Column 3* | *Column 4* |

VARIATIONS
There are a number of ways in which this game can be simplified or made easier for those with less ability. Draw a grid as shown in Appendix 13 on a board. Fill in appropriate categories and have the group shout out the answers. Alternatively, give out photocopies of Appendix 13 after dividing the group into small teams.

The categories can be made simple by choosing themes such as colours, flowers and so on, or more difficult by selecting categories such as chemicals, politicians or explorers. Easy or difficult letters of the alphabet may also be chosen. For example, W or J will be much more difficult than S or A. The list of categories can be added to the grid in Appendix 13 before photocopying.

COMMENT
This game is good fun and exercises quick recall.

Category Circle

MATERIALS Board (optional)

PREPARATION None

PROCEDURE
Form the group into a circle and call out a category, such as 'cities'. The person to your left states a city and then the next person gives another city. This continues around the circle until someone is unable to think of any new cities. When this happens, that person has to think of a new category, such as makes of cars, flowers, authors, types of cake, and so on. This then continues in the same way as before until someone else becomes stuck and thinks of another category.

VARIATION
Divide the group into teams. One team calls out a category and then it goes from team to team until one becomes stuck. When that happens, a new category is introduced, as before.

COMMENT
To help those who may have difficulty thinking of categories, either prepare a list or start the game by having group members shout them out and write them up on a board. If a player is unable to think of a category, they can then use one which has been written on the board.

This is another good quick recall game which provides a lot of fun. Although it is a similar game to 'Categories', some players find it more spontaneous and easier—and it does not need so much time.

What I Know About

MATERIALS Pieces of paper; board (optional); bag

PREPARATION
Write a different topic on each piece of paper. Examples:

Australia	training dogs	tennis	farming
America	growing tomatoes	flying kites	fishing
making curry	dancing	dieting	snooker
cricket	politicians	mountain climbing	

PROCEDURE
Put the pieces of paper into a hat or bag. Have a group member draw one out and read it aloud. Members of the group then contribute what they know about the subject until the whole group's knowledge about the topic has been shared. Encourage a lighthearted approach, asking group members to relate personal experiences. When one topic has been exhausted, have another group member draw another subject from the bag.

VARIATIONS
1 Have the group member who draws out the slip of paper give a one minute impromptu talk on the subject, beginning with the words: "What I know about…"
2 Have the group brainstorm topics. Write these up on a board as they are called out. Take the topics one at a time and encourage the group to share their knowledge on each one.
3 Instead of using a general mixture of subjects, stick to one theme, such as famous people, politicians, leisure activities, occupations, sports, countries and so on.

COMMENT
This exercise can stimulate a lot of personal memories as well as help participants to express knowledge about each topic.

Section Six

General Games

6

Some general memory and concentration games

Name Game

6

MATERIALS None

PREPARATION None

PROCEDURE
Have everyone sit in a circle. Request that a volunteer state their name and something about themselves that they do not mind sharing with the group. An example would be: "My name is Harry Campbell and I have four grandchildren." The player on his left now repeats what the first person has said, states their own name, and shares a personal detail with the group. The third person repeat the information given by the first and second players before stating their own name and personal detail. This procedure continues round the circle. The last person will have to remember everyone's name and details, but these will have been repeated numerous times.

DISCUSSION
After completing the circle, have a discussion about the different statements an information everyone has shared. Do group members share some experiences and values? Have they been actively involved in similar interests in the past?

VARIATION
The game can be made simpler by merely having everyone repeat the names of group members in this manner.

COMMENT
If players have difficulty remembering, clues can be given by other members of the group to act as a prompt. The discussion can be valuable for reminiscence purposes. The game is also a good introduction exercise to help familiarize eac player with others' names.

Autobiographies

MATERIALS None

PREPARATION None

PROCEDURE
Have each player choose a partner. Allow about five minutes for participants to
introduce themselves to their partners. Encourage them to help each other by
asking questions such as "Where were you born?", "Have you any hobbies?" and
"Which TV programmes do you like?" When the time is up, get everyone together
again in a circle and have each couple introduce their partner to the whole
group. Ensure that the person being introduced has an opportunity to put right
any details their partner may get wrong when doing the introduction.

DISCUSSION
When the introductions are completed, explore people's shared interests: places
lived, careers, places visited, and so on.

VARIATION
If the ability of the group allows, once the partners have introduced themselves
to each other, have each set of partners join another set, making a group of four.
Partners then introduce their companions, in turn, to the other two. When this
has been completed, partners then move on to form another group of four and go
through the process again. This continues until each player has had an
opportunity to be introduced to everyone else.

COMMENT
This is a good memory exercise which helps people to remember each other and
get to know others on a personal basis.

123

Ball Game

6

MATERIALS Soft ball or sponge

PREPARATION None

PROCEDURE
Have everyone sit in a circle. Pass the ball round the circle with everyone clearly stating their name as they hold it and before passing it on. This can be repeated if necessary, two or three times to ensure people become familiar with names. When the ball comes back to the beginning again, the group leader states the name of a group member, establishes eye contact with them and throws the ball to them. That person catches it and throws it back. The leader then states someone else's name and throws the ball to them. This continues until everyone has had their name called out a few times. Next, the group leader throws the ball to a group member who then calls out another player's name and throws the ball to them. That person then does the same. The game can then continue in this manner until everyone is thoroughly familiar with all names.

DISCUSSION
Repetition is a good way of remembering. How many of the group use the method to remember everyday things? What else do people remember by repetition? Poems, songs and so on? Have people recite the words of favourite poems and songs.

COMMENT
This game is fun, provides gentle exercise and helps with concentration as well as helping people to remember each other's names. It makes a good introduction or warm-up exercise, which can be stopped at any of its three stages, depending on the ability of group members.

Snowball Talk

MATERIALS

Pencils, paper, cassette and cassette-player or record and record player

PREPARATION   None

PROCEDURE

Stage 1

Ask the players to choose a partner, shake hands and introduce themselves. When they have done so, explain that the object is to find out as much as possible about each other in a few minutes. When the few minutes are up, start the music, at which time everyone must find a new partner. When the music stops, they will have another few minutes to shake hands and discover as much as possible about this new person. Tell them that the procedure will continue in this manner for a set period – 10 to 15 minutes is usually long enough – or until there has been sufficient opportunity for everyone to meet.

Stage 2

Sit everyone in a circle and give out pencils and paper. Ask each player to write down the names of everyone to whom they have spoken and what they can remember about each person. Allow a few minutes and then ask each player to read out what they have written. Give opportunities for group members to correct any details which are inaccurate.

DISCUSSION

The activity can end with a discussion on how difficult it is to remember the names of new people. How do various participants deal with this?

VARIATION

Have the initial partners form an inner and outer circle facing each other. When the music is playing, the inner circle moves to the right and the outer to the left. When the music stops, each player talks to the person opposite.
The game can be made more simple by asking players to remember names only.

▶ *125*

6 COMMENT

Using music gives an air of fun and relaxation to this game. Instead of players writing down what they remember, they can simply be asked to state what they remember, but, if members are able, the act of writing can help them to remember more and also to retain more.

Memory Cards

MATERIALS Cards, magazines with lots of pictures in them, pens, paper

PREPARATION
Cut out pictures from the magazines. Make these as different as possible: one could feature flowers, another a boat, the next a mountain scene, and so on. Paste each picture onto a card. How many cards you need will depend on the abilities of players, but 10 to 15 should be demanding enough for most groups.

PROCEDURE
Show one of the pictures to the group members. As you do so, invite comments about what is depicted. Discuss the colours and anything else relevant. Pass the picture around the players so that they can get a good look at it and make comments. When everyone is familiar with it, show them a second picture, discussing it in the same way. Continue in this manner until all the pictures have been passed around and discussed. Collect all the pictures and hand out pens and paper to players. Ask them to write down what they remember about as many pictures as they can recall. These can be brief descriptions, such as 'mountain scene', 'flowers' and so on, or more detailed. When this has been completed, go through the pictures, showing each one again, and see how many of them players have remembered.

VARIATIONS
Use fewer pictures, but ask players to draw what they remember about each one.
For more able groups, place the cards around the room and have them circulate to look at and discuss each picture.

COMMENT
The number of pictures can be adjusted to suit any group. Less able players can start with two to five pictures and then the number can be increased as they become more able.

Journalist

6 | **MATERIALS** Pens, paper

PREPARATION None

PROCEDURE

Stage 1

Divide the players into two groups and ask them to form two rows facing each other. If there are an equal number of men and women, make sure each player has a partner of the opposite sex. Explain that you want partners to make conversation, finding out as much as possible about each other in the three or four minutes allowed. Encourage players to ask each other questions and to volunteer information if partners become stuck.

Stage 2

When the time limit is up, send one group into another room. Give everyone a pen and a piece of paper. Ask them to pretend to be a journalist and write a short piece about their partner for the local paper. This will comprise a description and as much information derived from the previous conversation as possible.

Stage 3

Bring the two groups back together again and sit them in a circle. Have everyone, in turn, read out what they have written and see how observant they have been. Give the person being written about an opportunity to correct errors of memory and so on.

DISCUSSION

This is another game in which you can discuss things which group members have had in common, such as jobs, places lived, experiences and so on. You can also discuss the accuracy of the memories. What did they get wrong? What caused the errors? Did they hear incorrectly and did they not like to ask the person to repeat what they had said, misunderstand or feel too anxious to take the detail? Explore the difficulties and ways of dealing with them. If participant are anxious, learning to get their breathing rate right may help. If they are not sure that they heard something correctly, repeating it back to the other person will establish its accuracy.

COMMENT
It is important to give the players only enough instruction to complete one stage of this game at a time. If they are encouraged to make positive comments on appearance and character, this also helps in building self-confidence and self-esteem. This is a good observation and memory exercise.

Mock Reception

6 **MATERIALS** Pens, paper

PREPARATION None

PROCEDURE
Ask each member of the group to think of a job, hobby or interest they have had
in the past. Give a moment for thought and ask each person, in turn, to introduce
themselves to the group, stating their name and the job or pastime. Have them
explain a little about it. They can start their introduction with the words, for
example, "I am ... ..., carpenter." As the group member describes the thing they
did, ask the others to imagine the person doing it. They can imagine it like a
cartoon if they wish.

When everyone has introduced themselves, give out pens and paper. Ask
players to write down as many names and occupations or interests as they can
remember. When this has been completed, go through each name and check
whether everyone has got both the name and the job or interest correct.

DISCUSSION
Explore the above as a way of aiding memory when being introduced to new
people. Do any of the group use this method? Emphasize the importance of
seeing the individual doing the job or hobby. The picture imagined can be
exaggerated in the mind to make it more memorable.

Also, when the above exercise had been completed, the group can discuss any
shared hobbies or experiences of particular jobs they have done in the past.

COMMENT
As well as exploring a method of memorizing names, this game is useful as an
introduction exercise to help people remember each other's names.

Man in the Moon

MATERIALS Pens, paper (optional); drawing paper, pencils (optional)

PREPARATION
Make a list of words or phrases which can be used to stimulate memories.
Examples:

policeman	weddings	snow	happy days
rain	some good fortune	holidays	rock and roll
being in love	contentment	jealousy	
getting your own way			

PROCEDURE
Ensure that everyone is sitting comfortably in a circle. Tell everyone that you are going to call out a word or phrase and you would like them to think about the first thing that comes into their heads.

Call out the first word or phrase and then ask for a volunteer to share what has come to mind. Explore this and then ask another group member to share their memory. Continue in this manner until everyone has participated and then call out another word or phrase to begin the process again.

VARIATIONS
1 Give each player a pen and paper. Call out the word or phrase and ask everyone to write about what comes to mind. Allow five to ten minutes for writing and then ask each person to share what they have written with the group.
2 Give each player some drawing paper and a pencil. Ask them to draw their associated memory. When this has been completed, have each person show their drawing to the group and enlarge on what has been illustrated.

COMMENT
Some amazing memories can come out of this exercise.

Colour Choice

6 **MATERIALS** Board (optional)

PREPARATION None

PROCEDURE
Have the group sit in a circle. Ask each person to share with other players their favourite colour or colours. Elicit the sort of things they have chosen in the past in the particular colour: clothes, furniture, a car, decoration of a room and so on. Explore with each person the memories evoked by the colour.

VARIATION
Write a number of colours up on a board. Now ask a group member to chose one of the colours. Request that players think of a period in the past that to them relates to the colour. Give an opportunity for each player to share their period and the connection they make with the colour. When one colour has been exhausted, move on to another.

COMMENT
Colours can evoke very strong memories for some people.

Word Association

MATERIALS None

PREPARATION None

PROCEDURE
Everyone sits in a circle. One participant starts by stating a subject such as 'water'. The player on their left repeats the word and then mentions something that comes into their mind, suggested by the word. This could be 'boats'. The person to their left repeats 'water' and 'boats' and adds something else suggested to them by boats, which might be 'the sea'. And so the game continues round the circle, each player repeating what has been said previously and adding another association of their own. It is important to have participants react and make their statements as quickly as possible without too much thought.

VARIATIONS
1 Simplify by not having to repeat the previous words. Each player states only what they associate with the word given by the player before them. See how long the association chain can be kept going without faltering and then begin with a new word.
2 Have one participant state a word and then go round asking each group member to recount a memory associated with the word. When everyone has shared their memory, begin again with another word.

COMMENT
This is a memory exercise that is both stimulating and fun.

Seasonal Memories

6

MATERIALS None

PREPARATION None

PROCEDURE
Have the group sit in a circle. Ask players to think about a month of the year they particularly like or dislike. Now ask each person, in turn, to state the month they have chosen, why they like or dislike it and of what it reminds them. It may have been the month they got married, had an accident, won an award or achieved an ambition. Encourage group members to ask questions and help each individual explore their memory.

VARIATIONS
1 Ask group members to think of seasons they particularly like or dislike and explore particular memories linked to them.
2 Ask group members to think of birthdays, holidays, or anniversary celebrations they particularly remember and share them with the group.
3 Write different months of the year on slips of paper and place them in a bag. Have a player draw one slip from the bag and share a memory connected to that month. Encourage other group members to join in with their memories of the same month. When everyone has had an opportunity to share their memory, have another player choose another month from the bag.

COMMENT
This exercise can bring out many memories—happy, sad and humorous. Encourage the sharing of memories, but be sensitive to those which still cause pain.

Life Roles

MATERIALS   Board, chalk; paper, pens (optional)

PREPARATION   None

PROCEDURE
Have the group call out the different roles we all play during our lives and write them up on the board. This may include roles such as mother, father, teacher, daughter, son, carer, patient, brother, sister, cousin, grandparent, helper, employer, wife, husband, student, guardian, lover and so on. Now have group members, in turn, select a role which they played at some time in their life and share it with the group. Encourage the process by having everyone ask questions to help explore each person's experience.

DISCUSSION
When everyone has had an opportunity to share one role, explore the roles that people enjoyed most in general discussion. Which roles did people dislike most?

VARIATION
Have everyone write on a slip of paper their favourite role. Place the pieces of paper, folded, in a bag and ensure that they are well shaken. Now ask a player to draw one out and read it aloud. Group members try to guess who wrote that particular role. When the person has been correctly guessed or owns up, they relate their memory of the role. If a particular role was enjoyed by more than one member, they take turns to share their memory.

COMMENT
This exercise can evoke strong and spontaneous memories as well as stimulating the expression of opinions about the various roles experienced.

Story Chain

6

MATERIALS Pen, paper

PREPARATION None

PROCEDURE
Ask three participants to leave the room. While they are out the remaining members of the group put together a short story. This can be as comic or ridiculous as the group want to make it. Ensure that there are a number of incidents in the story. Get someone to write down a very brief outline of the story to aid memory.

Next, ask for a volunteer to relate the story using the notes. When this person is ready, ask one of the three participants who left the room to return. The volunteer now relates the story in as much detail as possible. When the story has been told, another person who left the room earlier is invited back. The story is then related to that person by the first person invited back into the room. The second person, in turn, relates the story, as they have been told it, to participant three who left the room, who then relates it to the whole group again. By this time the story will usually have undergone many changes and it will have become a source of amusement to the group. End by having the story retold in its original version, using the notes made to ensure accuracy.

DISCUSSION
How has the story changed? What caused the changes: mishearing, not understanding, making assumptions about details missed or just forgetting points? What was left out and what was added, and why did this happen? Discuss the importance of ensuring that what has been heard is understood.

VARIATIONS
Instead of making a story up, read out a fairly short story or article. Ensure that the piece has quite a lot of detail in it.

COMMENT

This game is good fun and can lead to helpful sharing of the difficulties of remembering and discussion on ways of assisting individuals to remember accurately.

Alphabet Game

6 **MATERIALS** Paper, pen, bag

PREPARATION
Write a letter of the alphabet on each piece of paper, avoiding the more difficult letters such as Z and X; alternatively, use letters from a *Scrabble* game, excluding the more difficult letters

PROCEDURE
Jumble the pieces of paper together and put them in a bag. Now invite a group member to draw out a letter. The letter is called out and group members recall as many proverbs or sayings as possible beginning with that letter. Examples for the letter T might be as follows:

The end justifies the means.
There is many a slip between cup and lip.
Turn over a new leaf.
Take care of the pence and the pounds will take care of themselves.
The leopard cannot change its spots.

When the group have recalled as many as they can, have another player select another letter. Continue in this manner for as long as is appropriate.

DISCUSSION
When proverbs are called out, before moving on to a new letter or at the end of the game, discuss whether players have found the proverbs to be true. Can anyone remember incidents from life which illustrate the truth of particular proverbs?

VARIATIONS
Have the participant drawing the letters out of the bag select two letters. This time players think of people they have known with these initials. These can be personal friends or famous people. Each person tells the group about the person with the initials.

COMMENT

This can, of course, be played as a team game. It is a good idea to have a book of proverbs handy to give prompts if required and to check the meanings.

Musical Quiz

6

MATERIALS Tape recorder and tapes, record-player and records, pencils, paper

PREPARATION

Obtain a wide selection of records or tapes which have been popular over the years. Include the widest possible range of tastes: classical and popular music. Record short extracts from each, leaving a short gap between each recording. Compile a list of questions concerning each recording, such as "What is the name of the piece?", "Who is the singer?" and "Who wrote the lyrics?". Make the questions as varied as possible. Information can usually be found on the record sleeve.

PROCEDURE

Seat the group so that everyone can hear clearly. Play the first recording and then ask the questions about it. Have the players write down the answers. Before continuing with the next recording, players can call out their answers. Alternatively, go through the complete quiz, then return to the beginning of the tape and replay each piece before people call out the answers they have written down. When answers are given, ensure that ample time is allowed to discuss each piece of music so that players can express their opinions and recall their memories of the time when it was popular.

DISCUSSION

End the game by giving each player an opportunity to state the types of music they have liked over the years. What are their favourite songs? Do these bring back particular memories of what was happening in their lives at that time? How has popular music changed over the years?

VARIATION

For some groups it may be sufficient to play a few recordings in full and ask some prepared questions, giving an opportunity to share memories of the time the record was popular. The activity can, of course, focus on particular decades, cover many years or just relate to the recent past. Instead of writing down answers, players can call them out as a group. The activity also makes a good team game.

COMMENT
Music can be a very powerful prompt to memory. It does take quite a lot of effort to make up several musical quizzes, but it is well worth while as they provide prompts to memory, and an opportunity for discussion and interaction. They can also be used time and time again with different groups.

Matching Pairs

6 **MATERIALS** Pens, paper

PREPARATION

Gather together two sets of identical pictures. These can be of people or objects and can be cut out of two copies of the same magazine or newspaper. It is better to keep to simple objects, such as a tree, a house or a yacht. It also makes it easier if the people used are well known. Trim the pictures so that they are all the same size and then number the back of each one.

PROCEDURE

Show the group each picture in turn. Give people enough time to observe what i in the picture, then place it, face down, on a low table which can easily be seen by the whole group. Next, give each person a pen and some paper and invite them to write down which are the matching numbers for the same pictures.

VARIATION

Ask one volunteer from the group to watch as you place the pictures. The volunteer then picks out the matching pairs. When this has been completed, invite another group member to do the same. Continue in this manner until everyone has had an opportunity to have a go.

COMMENT

Start the game with a small number of pairs – say six – and then progress to nine, 12, 15 and so on, depending on the group's abilities. If it is difficult to find identical pictures, use two sets of playing or picture cards. However, bear in min that, when you are working with a group, large pictures cut from magazines will be easier for everyone to see and identify.

Observation Quiz

MATERIALS   Pens, paper

PREPARATION   Make out a questionnaire. Here are some suggested questions:

1 What colour are your partner's eyes?
2 Are they wearing a ring or any other jewellery?
3 What type of footwear are they wearing?
4 What colour are their shoes?
5 What colour shirt/blouse are they wearing?
6 What colour is their hair?
7 Is their hair long or short?
8 Are they wearing glasses?
9 Are they taller or shorter than you?
10 What colour socks/stockings are they wearing?

PROCEDURE

Have the players line up in two teams facing each other. Ask participants to introduce themselves to the person opposite and exchange information about their past, interests and so on. Allow about three minutes and then have the teams turn back to back. Better still, have one team go into another room. The important thing is that no one looks at their opposite number from this point on. Now give each player a pen and a sheet of paper and the prepared list of questions (or call them out, allowing time between each question for the answer to be written down). When the questions have been completed, bring the teams back together as before, so all players can read out their answers and check their accuracy. Alternatively, form a circle and have the answers read out, giving the person being described a chance to correct any mistakes. The game can be played by dividing players into pairs, instead of teams.

DISCUSSION

How important is it to take an interest and observe in order to remember details? What difficulties do the group experience? Explore any methods used by the group to help with these.

▶   *143*

6 **VARIATION**

Allow the players to view a prepared room for a few minutes and then give them a questionnaire to answer.

COMMENT

If the partners are paired as male and female, you can make out a separate questionnaire to suit. This is a good observation and memory exercise which is fun and also excellent for helping people to get to know each other better.

Nicknames

MATERIALS Pens, paper, a bag or hat; board (optional)

PREPARATION None

PROCEDURE
Sit the group in a circle. Give each person a pen and a piece of paper. Ask them to recall a nickname or a pet name they have been given at some time in their lives. This could be when they were a child or at work; the name could be a favourite name given by a loved one or a friend. Ask each person to write the nickname down. When this has been done, collect the slips of paper and put them in a bag. Next, have a volunteer draw a name from the bag and read it out. See if the group members can guess to whom the nickname belongs. When the person has been identified, or has owned up, explore how they acquired the nickname. Encourage other group members to ask questions. Once the story has been told, have another player draw out the next nickname and proceed as before. Continue in this way until everyone has had an opportunity to share their nickname with the group.

DISCUSSION
End the game by opening up a discussion on unusual nicknames people have come across. The name may be attributed to famous people, friends or people known to group members during their lifetime. Encourage individuals to share memories about the nicknamed person.

VARIATIONS
Instead of getting people to write their nicknames down, have them call out the names and write these up on a board. Then explore each person's story in turn.

COMMENT
This game is fun and can stimulate many memories. Be sensitive to any names which could be unkind or cruel.

Mime Copy

6

MATERIALS   None

PREPARATION   None

PROCEDURE
Ask four volunteers to leave the room. While they are out, the group decides on a sequence of events to mime. Examples:

Washing an elephant at the zoo.
Getting up in the morning and making the bed.
Doing the washing and hanging it out.
Bathing the baby and putting it to bed.
Washing and polishing the car.
Cutting the grass and doing the gardening.

When the sequence of events has been decided, a member of the group practises doing the mime. When ready, one of the four volunteers is invited back and the mime is performed for that person. Volunteer No. 2 is then called in and the mime is performed by volunteer No. 1 from memory. Then No. 2 repeats the mime again for No. 3, and No. 3 for No. 4. By this time the sequence of events will have changed drastically. Invite the person who did the original mime to do again. Now ask each of the volunteers what they thought the sequence of events was meant to be.

DISCUSSION
End the game with a discussion on how the sequence of events changed with each mime. What caused this to happen? What methods can be used to help remember accurately?

COMMENT
This game is a lot of fun and can demonstrate many of the the difficulties encountered when trying to remember.

Chess Master

MATERIALS A draughts or chess set, a cloth, squared paper, pens

PREPARATION Set up a draughts or chess board with a game partly played

PROCEDURE
Place the draughts or chess board, covered with a cloth, on a table. When the group members are ready, remove the cloth and invite everyone to walk around the table and observe the position of the draughts or chess pieces. Allow enough time for everyone to have a good look. Ask the players to sit down again. Cover the board and hand out the squared paper and pens. Now ask each person to reproduce the pattern of the game pieces on the squared paper. When everyone has completed the task, remove the cloth again and see who has got the positions correct.

DISCUSSION
End the game by having those who remembered the most share any methods they found helpful in order to remember.

COMMENT
Vary the number of game pieces placed on the board, according to the abilities of the group. It is also a good idea initially to play the game with only a few pieces on the board. Then do it again with an increased number of pieces, and so on.

Appendices

Life Graph

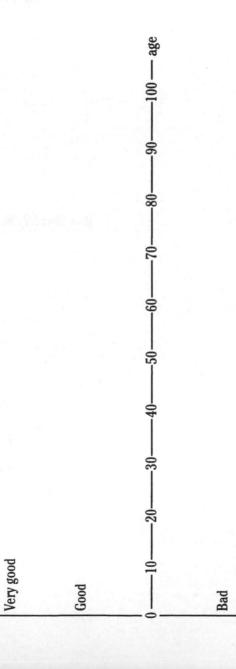

How was it?/Memorable Events

THE TWENTIES

1920 – Olympic Games held in Antwerp. **1921** – The first birth control clinic opened in London. **1922** – The first issue of *Readers' Digest* appeared. **1923** – Tokyo devastated by an earthquake. **1924** – Lenin, founder of Soviet Russia, died. **1925** – The 'Charleston' dance became popular. **1926** – Rudolph Valentino died. **1927** – Charles Lindbergh completed the first non-stop flight across the Atlantic, flying from New York to Paris. **1928** – Herbert C. Hoover elected President of the USA. **1929** – Black Thursday, the day Wall Street crashed.

THE THIRTIES

1930 – Unemployment in Britain broke the two million barrier. **1931** – Trolley buses began a regular service in London. **1932** – Charles Lindbergh's kidnapped baby was found in woods. **1933** – Hitler became Chancellor of Germany. **1934** – Fred Perry won the men's singles tennis championship at Wimbledon. **1935** – Malcolm Campbell smashed the 300mph barrier in 'Bluebird'. **1936** – Olympic Games held in Berlin. **1937** – The giant airship 'Hindenburg' exploded as she descended to land in New Jersey. **1938** – Walt Disney's first feature-length cartoon film, *Snow White and the Seven Dwarfs*, became a big success. **1939** – Britain declared war on Germany.

THE FORTIES

1940 – Allied forces evacuated from Dunkirk. **1941** – The pride of the German fleet, *Bismarck*, was sunk. **1942** – General Montgomery scored a triumph at El Alamein. **1943** – Humphrey Bogart and Claude Rains appeared in the film, *Casablanca*. **1944** – 'D-Day' landings in Normandy. **1945** – Germany surrendered. **1946** – Lord Mountbatten appointed Viceroy of India. **1947** – Princess Elizabeth and Prince Philip, Duke of Edinburgh, married.

1948 – Olympic Games held in London. **1949** – Wimbledon shocked by Gorgeou Gussie.

THE FIFTIES

1950 – Princess Anne born. **1951** – The Festival of Britain. **1952** – King George VI died. **1953** – Stiletto heels in fashion. **1954** – Roger Bannister ran a mile in under four minutes. **1955** – James Dean died in a car crash. **1956** – Grace Kelly married Prince Rainier III of Monaco. **1957** – The British prime minister, Harol Macmillan, said: "Let's be frank about it. Most of our people have never had it s good." **1958** – Some of the Manchester United football team were killed in a plane crash. **1959** – Charlton Heston starred in the film *Ben Hur*, which was to win 11 Oscars.

THE SIXTIES

1960 – The Russians shot down an American U2 aircraft piloted by Gary Power **1961** – Yuri Gagarin orbited the earth to become the first man in space. **1962** – The Brazilian football team won the World Cup. **1963** – John Kennedy shot dead in Dallas. **1964** – The Soviet leader, Nikita Khrushchev, ousted from power while on holiday. **1965** – The Beatles received MBEs at Buckingham Palace. **1966** – Richard Burton and Elizabeth Taylor starred in the film, *Who's Afraid of Virginia Wolf?* **1967** – Israel triumphed in the six day war against Arab states. **1968** – Martin Luther King shot dead. **1969** – Neil Armstrong became th first man to set foot on the moon.

THE SEVENTIES

1970 – France mourned the death of General de Gaulle. **1971** – Two astronauts went for a drive on the moon. **1972** – A band of 'Black September' Arab guerrill

broke into the Israeli building in the Olympic village near Munich, took hostages and demanded the release of 200 Palestinians held in Israeli jails.
1973 – Princess Anne married Captain Mark Phillips. **1974** – President Richard Nixon resigned the US presidency, facing impeachment for misdemeanours in the Watergate scandal. **1975** – Patty Hearst, the newspaper tycoon W.R. Hearst's granddaughter who was kidnapped and then became a 'guerrilla', was arrested on bank robbery charges. **1976** – The leader of Communist China, Mao Tse-tung, died. **1977** – Elvis Presley died. **1978** – Christopher Reeve starred in the film *Superman*. **1979** – Margaret Thatcher became Britain's first woman prime minister.

THE EIGHTIES

1980 – The British Special Air Service stormed the Iranian Embassy in London to free hostages. **1981** – Prince Charles and Lady Diana Spencer married. **1982** – Argentinians invaded the Falkland Islands. **1983** – Mother Teresa of Calcutta presented with the insignia of the Order of Merit by Queen Elizabeth II. **1984** – Jayne Torvill and Christopher Dean won an Olympic gold medal for ice dancing in Sarajevo. **1985** – Bob Geldof staged 'Live Aid' concerts in Wembley Stadium, London, and the JFK Stadium, Philadelphia. **1986** – Mike Tyson won the WBC world heavyweight boxing championship. **1987** – The car ferry, *Herald of Free Enterprise*, capsized outside the port of Zeebrugge. **1988** – George Bush elected president of the USA. **1989** – The Berlin Wall, the symbol of a divided world, came down.

Famous People

1920–1929

Vladimir Lenin	'Fatty' Arbuckle	Leon Trotsky
Woodrow Wilson	Mary Pickford	John Gilbert
Lloyd George	Enrico Caruso	Nellie Melba
Benito Mussolini	Franklin D. Roosevelt	Buster Keaton
Jack Dempsey	Sarah Bernhardt	Rudolph Valentino
Stanley Baldwin	Johnny Weissmuller	Eric Liddell
Bessie Smith	Josephine Baker	Joseph Stalin
Greta Garbo	Gabrielle 'Coco' Chanel	Al Jolson
Charles Lindbergh	Thomas Hardy	Isadora Duncan
Ronald Coleman	Lillie Langtry	George Bernard Shaw

1930–1939

Ramsay MacDonald	Helen Moody	Charlie Chaplin
Fred Perry	Noel Coward	Oswald Mosley
Shirley Temple	Fred Astaire	Mahatma Gandhi
Maurice Chevalier	Gracie Fields	Marlene Dietrich
Malcolm Campbell	Lawrence of Arabia	James Cagney
Jesse Owens	Edward VIII	Len Hutton
Mae West	W. C. Fields	Tyrone Power
Errol Flynn	Judy Garland	Amy Johnson
Al Capone	Jean Harlow	Joe Louis
Stan Laurel and	Margot Fonteyn	Clark Gable
Oliver Hardy		

1940–1949

John Buchan	Robert Taylor	Winston Churchill
Virginia Wolf	Vivien Leigh	Rudolf Hess
Ernest Bevin	Orson Wells	General Charles De Gaulle
Vera Lynn	James Joyce	Spencer Tracy
General Erwin Rommel	Bette Davis	Humphrey Bogart
Leslie Howard	Ingrid Bergman	Glenn Miller
Sergei Rachmaninov	Henry Moore	George Orwell
Christian Dior	Cary Grant	Lord Louis Mountbatten
Eva Peron	Freddie Mills	Don Bradman
General Dwight Eisenhower	Alec Guinness	Rita Hayworth

1950–1959

Frank Sinatra	Dylan Thomas	Bertrand Russell
Billy Graham	Randolph Turpin	Bill Haley
Gene Kelly	James Stewart	Maureen Connolly
Grace Kelly	Maria Callas	Albert Einstein
Albert Schweitzer	James Dean	Marilyn Monroe
Nikita Khrushchev	Edmund Hillary	Buster Crabbe
Sir Anthony Eden	Terry Spinks	Elvis Presley
Fidel Castro	Salvador Dali	Buddy Holly
Julie Andrews	Floyd Patterson	Raymond Chandler
Cliff Richard	Billie Holiday	Charlton Heston

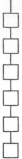

1960–1969

Anthony Perkins	Rod Laver	Alfred Hitchcock
Sonny Liston	John F. Kennedy	Peter O'Toole
Harold Wilson	Yuri Gagarin	Sean Connery
Rudolf Nureyev	Martin Luther King	Jomo Kenyatta
Elizabeth Taylor	Ian Smith	The Beatles
Lyndon B. Johnson	Sophia Loren	Ian Fleming
Leonid Brezhnev	Steve McQueen	Omar Sharif
Mick Jagger	Tom Jones	Rupert Murdoch
Richard Nixon	Golda Meir	Neil Armstrong
Cassius Clay (Muhammad Ali)	Tony Jacklin	Henry Cooper

1970–1979

George C. Scott	Henry Kissinger	Edward Heath
Woody Allen	Margaret Court	Pablo Picasso
Bobby Fischer	Moshe Dayan	Olga Korbut
W. H. Auden	Mark Spitz	Robert Redford
Alexander Solzhenitsyn	Chris Evert	Gerald Ford
John Conteh	John Curry	Niki Lauda
Bjorn Borg	Jimmy Carter	Sylvester Stallone
Virginia Wade	John Travolta	Daley Thompson
Andrew Lloyd Webber	Elaine Page	John Wayne
Ayatollah Khomeini	Agatha Christie	Dustin Hoffman

1980–1989

Ronald Reagan	Martina Navratilova	John McEnroe
Michael Jackson	Meryl Streep	Mikhail Gorbachev
Margaret Thatcher	Bruce Springsteen	Steven Spielberg
Boris Becker	Richard Attenborough	Madonna
David Niven	Diego Maradona	Mother Teresa
Shirley Maclaine	Jeffrey Archer	Andy Warhol
Mike Tyson	Anthony Hopkins	Lech Walesa
George Bush	Yasser Arafat	Alexander Dubcek
David Hockney	Salman Rushdie	Boris Yeltsin
Nelson Mandela	Luciano Pavarotti	Archbishop Desmond Tutu

Proverbs

1 All work and no play makes Jack a dull boy.

2 Every cloud has a silver lining.

3 First impressions are most lasting.

4 It is an ill wind that blows nobody any good.

5 Jack of all trades, master of none.

6 Love is blind.

7 Truth is stranger than fiction.

8 Give a fool enough rope and he will hang himself.

9 Fools rush in where angels fear to tread.

10 Everything comes to him who waits.

11 He who laughs best laughs last.

12 Listeners seldom hear good of themselves.

13 More haste, less speed.

14 Nothing ventured, nothing gained.

15 Practice makes perfect.

16 Pride goes before a fall.

17 Marry in haste; repent at leisure.

18 Forbidden fruit is sweetest.

19 When the cat is away the mice will play.

20 A fool and his money are soon parted.

Proverbs

1 All work and no play ...

2 Every cloud has ...

3 First impressions are ...

4 It is an ill wind that ...

5 Jack of all trades, ...

6 Love is ...

7 Truth is stranger ...

8 Give a fool enough rope and ...

9 Fools rush in where ...

10 Everything comes to ...

11 He who laughs best ...

12 Listeners seldom hear good ...

13 More haste, ...

14 Nothing ventured, ...

15 Practice makes ...

16 Pride goes before ...

17 Marry in haste; ...

18 Forbidden fruit is ...

19 When the cat is away ...

20 A fool and his money ...

Who Am I?

Princess Anne	Jayne Mansfield
Fred Astaire	P. G. Wodehouse
Harold Macmillan	Edward VIII
Archbishop Makarios	Gregory Peck
Queen Mary	Henry Fonda
Brigitte Bardot	Carroll Baker
Glenn Ford	Joan Crawford
Dean Martin	James Mason
Peter Sellers	Audrey Hepburn
Deborah Kerr	Dirk Bogarde
Bing Crosby	Paul Newman
Malcolm X	Lucille Ball
Robert Maxwell	Elton John
Doris Day	H. G. Wells
Diana Ross	Christiaan Barnard
Tony Jacklin	Alexander Fleming
Sigmund Freud	Roger Bannister
Billie Jean King	Louis Armstrong
Jerry Lewis	Tony Curtis
Marlon Brando	Paul Getty
Queen Elizabeth, the Queen Mother	Howard Hughes
Rock Hudson	Gary Cooper
General Montgomery	Lester Piggott
Cole Porter	Henry Ford
Nat King Cole	Ella Fitzgerald

True or False

1   During the Second World War people in Britain often used carrots instead of fruit when making Christmas puddings.

    ANSWER   True.

2   Canada's Ben Johnson was disqualified from the 1988 Seoul Olympic games after winning a gold medal.

    ANSWER   True. He was found guilty of using drugs.

3   'Little Mo' (Maureen Connolly) was only 17 years old when she won her first world swimming championship in 1952.

    ANSWER   False. She won the women's singles tennis championship at Wimbledon.

4   In 1962 Sonny Liston beat Floyd Patterson to become heavyweight boxing champion of the world.

    ANSWER   True.

5   In 1963 Jack Ruby shot President John Kennedy.

    ANSWER   False. Lee Harvey Oswald shot the president. Jack Ruby subsequently shot Oswald.

6   The American actor John Wayne appeared in many films but never won an Oscar.

    ANSWER   False. He won an Oscar for *True Grit*, in which he played a one-eyed US marshal.

161

7 In 1976, in a brilliant feat of arms, Israeli commandos flew 2500 miles and rescued over 100 hostages held at Entebbe airport in Uganda by pro-Palestinian skyjackers.

ANSWER True.

8 Yoko Ono married Paul McCartney in 1969.

ANSWER False. She married John Lennon.

9 Rudolph Valentino was 72 years old when he died in 1926.

ANSWER False. He was only 31 years old.

10 Adolf Hilter left the Berlin Olympic stadium in 1936 to avoid having to shake hands with the black athlete and gold medal winner, Jesse Owens.

ANSWER True.

11 In 1983 the Soviet Union shot down a Korean Airlines Boeing 747, on a flight from New York to Seoul, as it flew over the Sakhalin Islands off Siberia, with the loss of some 269 lives.

ANSWER True.

12 Harry Houdini, the great escapologist, died in 1926 while trying to escape from under ice in a frozen river.

ANSWER False. He died from peritonitis after the removal of his appendix at the age of 52.

13 The American star Rock Hudson died in 1985 after a fatal accident.

ANSWER False. He died after a battle with AIDS.

14 Rudolf Hess, Hitler's trusted deputy, was found in a field in Scotland in 1941 by a ploughman.

ANSWER   True. He said he had an important message for the Duke of Hamilton.

15 The nuclear reactor disaster at Chernobyl in the Ukraine in 1986 was initiated by sabotage.

ANSWER   False.

16 The giant airship 'Hindenburg' was shot down by a sniper as she came in to land in New Jersey in 1937.

ANSWER   False. The airship exploded in a ball of fire. The cause was unknown but it was believed to have been static electricity.

17 In her forties, the child star Shirley Temple took up a second career in public life as an ambassader for the USA.

ANSWER   True.

18 Paul Newman starred with Meryl Streep in the film *Out of Africa* in 1985.

ANSWER   False. It was Robert Redford.

19 In 1960 a British court ruled that D. H. Lawrence's novel, *Lady Chatterley's Lover*, was obscene.

ANSWER   False. The court ruled that it was not obscene.

20 In 1978 Patrick Swayze starred in the musical *Grease*.

ANSWER   False. It was John Travolta.

People Categories

Category	1	2	3

Jumbled Novelists

	Novel	Novelist	Answer
1	The Heart of the Matter	HAMARG NEEGRE	
2	Wuthering Heights	MILYE ETRONB	
3	Death on the Nile	ATHAGA HCISRIET	
4	Gone with the Wind	MGARAETR LLCHEIMT	
5	Pride and Prejudice	NEAJ ENTUSA	
6	To Kill a Mockingbird	HPARRE EEL	
7	A Passage to India	E. M. ORTSERF	
8	The Grapes of Wrath	NJHO TNEISCKEB	
9	Robinson Crusoe	ANDEIL EFDOE	
10	Of Human Bondage	MOSSREET GHMAAUM	
11	The Catcher in the Rye	J. D. LANIGRES	
12	Death in Venice	MOSATH NNMA	
13	An American Dream	NAMORN IALREM	
14	Rebecca	PHENDA UD AUMRRIE	
15	Frankenstein	YRMA LLHESEY	
16	A Farewell to Arms	NESTRE MEHGINYAW	

17 Lady Chatterley's Lover   D. H. RECENWAL   _____

18 Dr Zhivago   ROISB TERKANASP   _____

19 The Young Lions   IRNIW WASH   _____

20 Great Expectations   LARESCH IKCNSED   _____

21 A Town Like Alice   VEINL HUSET   _____

22 The Carpetbaggers   HLDROA BORNIBS   _____

23 The Good Companions   J. B. IETSEYLPR   _____

24 The Thirty Nine Steps   HONJ UHCNAB   _____

25 The Great Gatsby   TOCST TIFGZRAEDL   _____

26 The Time Machine   H. G. LELWS   _____

27 Portnoy's Complaint   ILPIHP HTOR   _____

28 The Day of the Jackal   EDRERFKCI ROYSHTF   _____

29 Babbitt   NISLCIAR WELIS   _____

30 The Call of the Wild   JCKA NODONL   _____

Jumbled Novelists

ANSWERS

1 Graham Greene
2 Emily Bronte
3 Agatha Christie
4 Margaret Mitchell
5 Jane Austen
6 Harper Lee
7 E. M. Forster
8 John Steinbeck
9 Daniel Defoe
10 Somerset Maugham
11 J. D. Salinger
12 Thomas Mann
13 Norman Mailer
14 Daphne du Maurier
15 Mary Shelley
16 Ernest Hemingway
17 D. H. Lawrence
18 Boris Pasternak
19 Irwin Shaw
20 Charles Dickens
21 Nevil Shute
22 Harold Robbins
23 J. B. Priestley
24 John Buchan
25 Scott Fitzgerald
26 H. G. Wells
27 Philip Roth
28 Frederick Forsyth
29 Sinclair Lewis
30 Jack London

Jumbled Film Stars

	Film	Film Star	Answer
1	Citizen Kane	OSRNO LLESW	
2	Yankee Doodle Dandy	MESJA GNEYCA	
3	The Outlaw	AENJ RSSLLEU	
4	The Lost Weekend	AYR LLDANIM	
5	The Paleface	BBO OPHE	
6	Samson and Delilah	TROCIV URTEAM	
7	The Wizard of Oz	UDJY LRADNAG	
8	The African Queen	THRANEIKA HPBEUNR	
9	Singin' in the Rain	NEEG LLEYK	
10	Limelight	LEIRAHC HCAPNIL	
11	Niagara	MLIRAYN ONEORM	
12	The Glenn Miller Story	MESAJ SEWTTAR	
13	From Here to Eternity	ANRKF SATARIN	
14	The King and I	BEDORHA RRKE	
15	The Ten Commandments	ARLNOTHC SETNOH	
16	The Bridge On The River Kwai	CEAL GNNSSUIE	

17	The Nun's Story	DYERUA PBEHRNU
18	Psycho	ATHNNYO KNISERP
19	The Guns of Navarone	DAVDI NNEVI
20	Lolita	MESAJ NOSMA
21	The Great Escape	TSVEE QEEUNcM
22	Goldfinger	EANS NNYREOC
23	The Graduate	INTUSD FFNAMHO
24	The Godfather	NOLARM ONARDB
25	Jaws	RTEOBR WASH
26	The Omen	ROYGREG KPCE
27	Indiana Jones	RRAHSINO DORF
28	On Golden Pond	RNYEH ADFNO
29	Fatal Attraction	NNLGE LOESC
30	The Silence of the Lambs	IEDOJ TSREOF

Jumbled Film Stars

ANSWERS

1 Orson Wells
2 James Cagney
3 Jane Russell
4 Ray Milland
5 Bob Hope
6 Victor Mature
7 Judy Garland
8 Katharine Hepburn
9 Gene Kelly
10 Charlie Chaplin
11 Marilyn Monroe
12 James Stewart
13 Frank Sinatra
14 Deborah Kerr
15 Charlton Heston
16 Alec Guinness
17 Audrey Hepburn
18 Anthony Perkins
19 David Niven
20 James Mason
21 Steve McQueen
22 Sean Connery
23 Dustin Hoffman
24 Marlon Brando
25 Robert Shaw
26 Gregory Peck
27 Harrison Ford
28 Henry Fonda
29 Glenn Close
30 Jodie Foster

Geography Quiz

1   Into which sea does the river Danube flow?

2   Which province of Canada has a large French-speaking population?

3   Of which country is Kuala Lumpur the capital?

4   In which American state would you find Long Island?

5   In which country would you find the Transvaal?

6   Which country would you be in if you lived and worked in a kibbutz?

7   What is the capital of Denmark?

8   If you lived in Valencia, which country would you be in?

9   In which country are the Cambrian Mountains?

10 Which sea surrounds the island of Jamaica?

11 In which capital city would you find Vatican City?

12 In which capital city would you find Trafalgar Square?

13 On which country's borders would you find the Victoria Falls?

14 Which continent has the largest land area?

15 What is the capital of Vietnam?

16 In which country would you be if you were standing on the Giant's Causeway?

17 In which country is the Taj Mahal?

18 What is the largest desert in the world?

19 In which country would you be if you were viewing the Pyramids?

20 In which city would you find Red Square?

Geography Quiz

ANSWERS

1 The Black Sea
2 Quebec
3 Malaysia
4 New York
5 South Africa
6 Israel
7 Copenhagen
8 Spain
9 Wales
0 Caribbean (Atlantic Ocean also acceptable)
1 Rome
2 London
3 Zimbabwe and Zambia border (formerly Southern and Northern Rhodesia)
4 Asia
5 Hanoi
6 Northern Ireland
7 India
8 Sahara
9 Egypt
0 Moscow

Jumbled Places

1	EYRKTU	_____	16	ONDONL	_____
2	AGOCIHC	_____	17	HNSTAE	_____
3	LANAIDTH	_____	18	VEROUNCVA	_____
4	RABLECNOA	_____	19	TANISLUB	_____
5	WCOOSM	_____	20	ASLLAD	_____
6	LNIBDU	_____	21	USLAMEREJ	_____
7	MBOAYB	_____	22	ANVAAH	_____
8	ERLNIB	_____	23	CIAOR	_____
9	ATSMDAEMR	_____	24	MOCXIE	_____
10	RSIAP	_____	25	OGHN NGOK	_____
11	MAHRGBU	_____	26	ENVCIE	_____
12	ONTOROT	_____	27	APEC NWTO	_____
13	YNDYES	_____	28	EMRO	_____
14	ASOWGLG	_____	29	BMELUONER	_____
15	SHWANGIONT	_____	30	ALCCTTAU	_____

Jumbled Places

ANSWERS

1	Turkey	11	Hamburg	21	Jerusalem
2	Chicago	12	Toronto	22	Havana
3	Thailand	13	Sydney	23	Cairo
4	Barcelona	14	Glasgow	24	Mexico
5	Moscow	15	Washington	25	Hong Kong
6	Dublin	16	London	26	Venice
7	Bombay	17	Athens	27	Cape Town
8	Berlin	18	Vancouver	28	Rome
9	Amsterdam	19	Istanbul	29	Melbourne
10	Paris	20	Dallas	30	Calcutta

Categories

Category	Initial letter:	Initial letter:	Initial Letter

Alphabetical List of Games

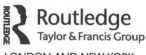